Caring for someone with arthritis

Jim Pollard

BOOKS

Published by Age Concern England
1268 London Road
London SW16 4ER

First published 2000

Editor   Gillian Clarke
Production   Vinnette Marshall
Designed and typeset by GreenGate Publishing Services, Tonbridge, Kent
Printed in Great Britain by Bell & Bain Ltd, Glasgow

A catalogue record for this book is available from the British Library.

ISBN 0–86242–266–3

Bulk orders
Age Concern England is pleased to offer customised editions of all its titles to UK companies, institutions or other organisations wishing to make a bulk purchase. For further information, please contact the Publishing Department at the address on this page. Tel: 020 8765 7200. Fax: 020 8765 7211. E-mail: addisom@ace.org.uk.

Contents

About the author

Jim Pollard is a writer and editor. He writes for national newspapers and magazines, primarily on health issues, and extensively for the Department of Health. Jim has also worked for some of the UK's leading voluntary organisations, including Arthritis Care where he was editor of *Arthritis News* and subsequently Director of Communications.

He is author of three health books, including *Getting A Grip – Self-help for arthritis and rheumatism* (Headline 1996) and the acclaimed *All Right, Mate – An easy introduction to men's health* (Vista 1999). His novel *Rotten in Denmark* was published in 1999.

Acknowledgements

Thanks very much to all the people with arthritis whose ideas and insights have informed this book and to all the carers too. Some are named in the book but many more are not or have had their names changed. Thanks also to everybody at Age Concern and Arthritis Care, both staff and volunteers, who helped put this book together. I am very grateful to Arthritis Care for their continued support and for permission to quote from their publications in this book.

Particular acknowledgement, in no particular order, is due to Margaret Stephens and the Kings and Dulwich branch of Arthritis Care; to Richard Holloway and Evelyn McEwen at Age Concern; to the information and counselling team and publications department at Arthritis Care; to my mum and dad, June and David Pollard; to Gillian Clarke for her patient and thorough editing; to Richard Gutch, Jean Ashcroft, Roy Jones, Dr D John Dickson, Penny Boot and Kate Nash for their invaluable advice and comment; to Bela Maria for putting up with my moaning; and to my agent, Amanda White.

Introduction

This book is aimed at anyone who is or is considering caring for a person with arthritis and wondering whether it is the best way ahead for you both. It gives basic information about arthritis and how it is treated, and raises some of the practical and personal issues you will need to think about if you are to care for somebody with the disease.

Both of you will probably want to read the book, because, as far as possible, it should always be the person being cared for who makes the decisions about their life. That is easily said but hard to do. It's just one of the challenges that caring brings.

I have not been a carer myself but I have seen in my own family the impact that caring and the need for care can have. My personal experience is in working with people with arthritis – for five years I worked for the charity Arthritis Care. I have discussed caring and carers with many disabled people with care needs and it is mainly their views that inform this book. This is not to say that the views of carers are secondary, because I have spoken to many carers too. But when you are considering whether to become a carer, it is important also to bear in mind the views of the person who will be receiving your care.

Whatever you decide, caring is not something that you should drift into – it should be the result of a considered decision. You may find that you have become a carer gradually over time and now want to consider the options that are open to you both. I hope this book will help you make a choice.

1 What is arthritis?

This chapter gives a broad overview of the six main categories of arthritis. There then follows more detailed information on the common types, with emphasis on osteoarthritis and rheumatoid arthritis.

Unless you have arthritis, it can sometimes be difficult to understand the problems that the condition can bring, so the chapter includes comments from people saying what it is like for them. Of course, everyone is different, and the person you are caring for will not necessarily agree with all the views expressed, but this helps to emphasise just how important it is to discuss the issues that arthritis raises.

Joy

'I got arthritis in 1972 as the result of a road traffic accident, a car crash. I suffered disc compression in the spine and my walking was affected. However, at first they put my subsequent problems down to stress from the accident.

'I was working as a nurse then on a children's fracture ward, but even so it seemed like the end of the world. It's the not knowing. If you don't know what's happening, you can't come to terms with it and move forward.

'While I was still off sick after the accident, I was sent to a rehabilitation unit where the doctor said there was more wrong than I'd been told. I've a lot to thank him for. He sent me to a rheumatology unit. All in all, it took 18 months before my arthritis was diagnosed.

'A lot of problems are caused by other people's attitudes. I don't want sympathy and I don't want to be patronised ... I could have knocked the block off one rheumatologist! Now I'm better able to talk to doctors but it's only come with experience. I usually know more about arthritis than they do.'

From Getting a Grip: Self-help for arthritis *by Jim Pollard; Headline 1996*

What arthritis is

Two myths about arthritis

One of the great myths about arthritis is that it affects only older people. In fact, according to Arthritis Care and the Arthritis Research Campaign, arthritis is the major cause of physical disability in the UK, affecting 8 million people – including about 15,000 children. One million people with arthritis are under 45 years of age and a further 3 million under 65. Put another way, one in twenty people under 45 has arthritis, more than one in five between 45 and 65 and more than two in five over 65. This means that carers of people with arthritis come in all ages, too.

The second great myth about arthritis is that it is trivial. Because it is so widespread, because nobody will die from arthritis alone and because everyone knows someone who has it, even if it's only the family pet, people assume that it is not serious. Unless you yourself have the disease, it is often very hard to appreciate just how difficult it can be and in how many ways.

The media tend to present two contrasting images of arthritis. The first reinforces the view that it is something trivial that happens only to older people. The second, arising out of the media's general stereotype of disabled people, is rather the opposite: that it is something terrible that leaves you in a wheelchair and dependent. These images are confusing. And inaccurate. Arthritis is rarely trivial, but using a wheelchair does not mean giving up your independence.

Professionals in the health and social services, who should know better, can be as guilty of falling for these myths as the rest of us. When you care for someone with arthritis, you have the additional challenges of trying to get the disease taken seriously and, in some cases, getting it believed at all.

An overview of arthritis

The name 'arthritis' comes from the Greek *arthron* meaning 'joint' and *itis* meaning 'inflammation'. There are as many as 100 different types of the disease, and it is a feature of about 100 other diseases. Some types of arthritis do not feature inflammation but all involve the joints. You will hear different terms used. Some doctors talk of rheumatic or musculo-skeletal disorders; some patients talk about their rheumatism. They are all talking about what this book calls arthritis. The disease is caused by a number of factors but exactly how and why are still far from fully understood by medical science. Nevertheless, you don't need detailed knowledge about the condition to care for someone with arthritis.

The one thing that can be said with certainty is that arthritis is different for everyone who has it. It is always important to listen to the patient, whatever the disease, but in arthritis it is more important than most. The information in this book is for guidance only. Don't be surprised if the person you are caring for doesn't fit neatly into any of the categories discussed here.

There are six broad categories of arthritis:

- *Osteoarthritis* – disease in which the cartilage at the joint wears away, leaving bone rubbing against bone.

3

■ *Inflammatory* – diseases that begin with swelling in the synovial membrane (the inner lining of the capsule around a movable joint and the tendon sheaths), which contains synovial fluid that lubricates a joint or moving tendon. For example, rheumatoid arthritis.

■ *Periarticular* – diseases that occur outside the joint, where the tendons and ligaments join the bone. For example, ankylosing spondylitis.

■ *Crystal* – diseases that result from crystals forming in the joint. For example, gout.

■ *Infective* – diseases arising from viruses or bacteria in the joint (or, sometimes, the gut), called reactive arthritis. For example, Reiter's disease.

■ *Muscular* – diseases of the muscle. Although not strictly speaking forms of arthritis, the symptoms and the experiences of people with these conditions can be similar. For example, fibrositis and polymyalgia rheumatica.

Osteoarthritis

Osteoarthritis is the most common form of arthritis. Estimates by doctor and patient organisations suggest that as many as 3 million people in the UK have it severely enough to discuss it with their GP. Many others have it in a milder form. After heart disease it is the single major cause of disability in adults.

There is a close relationship between age and osteoarthritis: one American study estimated that 85 per cent of people aged 75–79 have osteoarthritis compared with just 4 per cent in the 18–24 age group. Most people over 65 have one or more joints with moderate to severe osteoarthritis: it becomes more common as we age, especially if we do not look after our joints through appropriate use and exercise. Nevertheless, the disease is not simply the inevitable result of ageing, and can affect anyone of any age at any time.

Generally, osteoarthritis develops slowly. The cartilage becomes worn and bony lumps form, which can make the joint look knobbly.

Later the bones begin to rub together. This stage can be very painful and cause the joint to change shape.

Osteoarthritis most commonly affects the knees, hips, hands, feet and spine. Because of its many, often tiny, joints – there are over 150 – the spine is particularly vulnerable, with the neck (the cervical region) and the lower back (the lumbar region) most usually affected.

The hips are more usually affected in men, the knees in women – which may say something about the traditional working roles of the sexes. Because of the use to which these joints are subjected, osteoarthritis in the hip and knee may well worsen more quickly than in other joints, some of which can remain relatively unchanged for years.

Although the synovial membrane may become inflamed in some cases, the term osteoarthritis is not particularly accurate because inflammation is not generally involved. Unlike some other types of arthritis, osteoarthritis is not usually a systemic disease (affecting the whole body), it is joint specific. Sites of old sports injuries, for example, are particularly vulnerable. The typical causes of neck pain are good examples of the two ways osteoarthritis problems develop. They may arise from a particular incident – a whiplash injury, for example, in a car accident – or they may develop over a longer period – the result of an awkward sleeping position, poor posture or working position or a combination of all these and more.

Osteoarthritis varies considerably from person to person. Some people with the early stages of osteoarthritis may never realise they have it, whereas others find it very disabling and may eventually need surgery. Because so many people are affected with joint pains, it can be difficult to get osteoarthritis taken seriously even by those who should know better. At its most severe, osteoarthritis is a very painful and disabling condition.

It is important to get osteoarthritis properly diagnosed. Don't be fobbed off with vague talk about 'a natural sign of ageing' or 'the symptoms are difficult to observe clinically'. You need to know if it is osteoarthritis because it will be crucial to get the right balance between rest and exercise. Joints affected by osteoarthritis tend to be more painful at the end of the day and after exercise. On the other hand, they will become stiff if left inactive. Getting the balance right can make the difference between being in control of the disease and being controlled by it.

Rheumatoid arthritis

Rheumatoid arthritis, the most common type of inflammatory arthritis, is more prevalent than one might imagine. This is because, as with osteoarthritis, it can go unnoticed in its early stages. According to Arthritis Care and the Arthritis Research Campaign, about 1 per cent of the population – 600,000 people in the UK – have what rheumatologists call 'definite' rheumatoid arthritis, but perhaps as many as 1 million people have it to some degree.

These facts are important because, although there is some evidence that the incidence and severity of rheumatoid arthritis are decreasing, the longer life expectancy of people in general and of people with rheumatoid arthritis in particular means that there will be more older people with rheumatoid arthritis in the years to come. Today's older people with long-term disabilities brought on by rheumatoid arthritis are among the first. This is another reason to listen to what they say about their experiences.

Rheumatoid arthritis usually begins in the hands and feet. It generally comes on in relatively early life – before the age of 40 – but people in their 70s and 80s may also develop the condition. It affects three times as many women as men.

The disease occurs as the body's immune system malfunctions. Instead of protecting the body as it should, the immune system turns on it and attacks it. Inflammation, which is a good thing when the auto-immune system is working properly (a sign that the body is successfully repelling invaders), becomes an enemy within. These attacks can be severe – the immune system tends to shoot first and ask questions later. Inflammation of the synovial membrane around the joint causes damage to the ligaments, tendons, cartilage and the joint itself.

It is not only the joints that are affected in rheumatoid arthritis, it is the whole body. Debilitating tiredness and aching muscles, similar to a severe bout of flu, are very common. The eyes, skin and, in a few cases, other organs, may also be affected. For this reason, rheumatoid arthritis is often referred to as rheumatoid *disease*. Blood tests are commonly used to aid diagnosis.

The disease may appear suddenly – this is more common in older people – or it may come on slowly – the more likely pattern in younger people. It gradually affects more joints over a period of months or it may be what doctors call 'palindromic', flaring up and easing again intermittently before finally setting in. These flareups, or flares, are also common in active rheumatoid arthritis.

In contrast with osteoarthritis, rheumatoid arthritis tends to affect the joints in a symmetrical way – both hands, both hips, both knees or both feet. Joint stiffness is more likely in the morning than in the evening.

In about one-third of cases of rheumatoid arthritis, the disease is fairly mild and does not cause severe long-term problems. Another third of patients will be moderately affected, and a further third will have what doctors term more 'aggressive' disease. At the point of diagnosis, it can be difficult to be certain into which category an individual will fall. However, doctors should try to assess this, because there is evidence that early and perhaps heavy drug intervention can reduce the likelihood of more severe disability later. What is more, most joint damage from rheumatoid arthritis occurs in the first two or three years, so early treatment is vital.

One way of estimating the likely development of the disease is through a blood test. Although it is not found in everybody with rheumatoid arthritis, there is some evidence that people with a particular protein in their blood – called rheumatoid factor – may go on to develop more severe rheumatic disease. (For more about rheumatoid factor, see p 24.)

Today's researchers are very interested in the way the immune system works and the way the body deals with inflammation. However, the immune system is an incredibly complex one and researchers stress that it will be a long time before they know whether their current approaches will be successful. You should take any medical breakthrough story you hear about in the media with a pinch of salt. In the case of arthritis, make it an especially large pinch!

Other types of arthritis

Ankylosing spondylitis

This may be the most difficult to pronounce of all the forms of arthritis but is actually very appropriately named. *Ankylosing* is from the Greek for 'stiffness' while *spondylitis* means 'inflammation of the spine'. After osteoarthritis and rheumatoid arthritis, ankylosing spondylitis is the third most common rheumatic disorder in the UK – affecting about 115,000 people, according to the Arthritis Research Campaign.

The disease affects more men than women – the ratio may be as high as five to one – and the usual age of onset is the late teens or early twenties. It usually starts in the lower back, the inflammation going on to cause the formation of bony scar tissue between the vertebrae. Untreated, this tissue will eventually fill the space between the bones and become bone itself, causing the joint to become rigid. This locking of the spine can be prevented by prompt diagnosis and treatment (the usual treatment is exercise). Over the years, the pain and stiffness tend to come and go, often disappearing completely by the age of 55 or 60.

Gout

Because its cause is precisely known, an attack of gout can be readily cured.

For most of us the uric acid in our blood is passed in our urine. Sometimes, however, for reasons that are not fully understood, crystals of uric acid can grow in the cartilage or joint space and the inflammation that results causes the swelling of gout. It usually affects the feet, especially the big toe, the ankles, hands and wrists. An attack, although lasting only a few days, can be very painful and may damage the cartilage.

Drugs and diet can reduce the amount of uric acid in the body. Losing weight may also help. If anti-inflammatory drugs are used, aspirin should be avoided because it can increase the level of uric acid.

Contrary to popular belief, gout is not caused by excess food or drink. However, certain types of either can make matters worse:

- **Food**: game; pâté; offal (liver, sweetbreads and kidney); some fish (shellfish, fish roe, salmon, herring and whitebait); yeast and its extracts; strawberries; rhubarb; spinach; and asparagus.
- **Drink**: port; and carbonated drinks, including beer, champagne and sparkling wine.

Lupus

Although it is treatable by rheumatologists, systemic lupus erythematosus (usually called 'SLE' or simply 'lupus') is not, strictly speaking, a type of arthritis. Rather, arthritis is a symptom of lupus, which is a disease of the auto-immune system. There is joint and muscle pain, fever and flu-like symptoms. Like rheumatoid arthritis, lupus can be mild or severe, and an up-and-down affair over the years, flaring up and then easing off. Sunlight (or even ultraviolet light from fluorescent lights) can sometimes trigger a flare-up in affected people.

Lupus is rare but seems to be increasing. Traditional estimates put the number of people with SLE in the UK at around 4,000 but this is generally thought by health professionals and patient organisations to be an under-estimate. The Arthritis Research Campaign suggest that 15,000 is a closer figure. Doctors are getting better at detecting the disease and this alone may explain the increase. They are also getting better at treating it, with the result that, although lupus remains a serious systemic disease, it is seldom fatal.

It affects far more women than men – the ratio is eight or nine to one – and is most common among women of child-bearing age.

Although the joints are painful, they are rarely damaged. The tendons, the skin and, in some cases, other organs of the body may become inflamed, particularly the kidneys. This inflammation can cause pains that may not at first seem obviously related to lupus. For example, chest pains may be the result of inflammation in the lungs.

Reactive arthritis

Arthritis can occur as a result of an infection, although it may not be immediately obvious that this is what has happened. Six weeks or so may elapse between the infection appearing and the subsequent joint inflammation. It is important to appreciate that, even after the infection has cleared up, arthritis may still remain or, indeed, appear for the first time. This type of arthritis is 20 times more common in men than in women.

The arthritis does not generally last very long, usually going into remission after a few months. A characteristic is that it moves around from one joint to another. Larger joints are most commonly affected – the knee, elbow or ankle are typical – and it rarely hits both of a pair of joints. Sometimes tendons become inflamed.

Two main types of infection can lead to reactive arthritis. One is the infection of the bowel with _Salmonella_ or a similar germ – the type that usually results in food poisoning. The second is a sexually transmitted infection. Most sexually transmitted diseases (STDs) can cause arthritis. The commonest is the 'non-specific urethritis' caused by the _Chlamydia_ organism. Arthritis may also appear as a complication of an infection elsewhere in the body, such as chickenpox or mumps.

In reactive arthritis, inflammation occurs in the synovial membrane around the joints and may be more painful in the morning.

Reiter's disease is a type of reactive arthritis in which inflammation also occurs in the eye (resulting in conjunctivitis or irisitis).

Psoriatic arthritis (psoriatic arthropathy)

The skin disease psoriasis – from the Greek word for 'itch' – is fairly common, usually affecting the elbows, knees and scalp. The skin becomes inflamed and red, and can seem scaly. It is not contagious and has nothing to do with an individual's personal hygiene.

A skin cell usually lives for a month or so, working its way to the skin's surface where it simply flakes off. Psoriatic cells pack all their activity into a week, dragging live cells with them to the skin's surface and causing a rash.

Arthritis is present in about 5 per cent of psoriasis cases, which means that about 30,000 people in the UK have psoriatic arthritis. It is not, strictly speaking, a single disease. Psoriasis accompanies a number of types of arthritis. It can appear, seemingly by coincidence, in rheumatoid arthritis. It can also appear with ankylosing spondylitis. Or it may signify another type of arthritis entirely. The exact connection is unclear but all conditions feature inflammation and a tendency to wax and wane over time.

Sjögren's syndrome

This is another type of auto-immune condition, and affects mostly middle-aged and post-menopausal women. In Sjögren's syndrome the immune system prevents the exocrine glands (eg the saliva and sweat glands) from properly secreting their substances. It results in dry eyes and dry mouth, and is usually accompanied by inflammatory arthritis – such as rheumatoid arthritis or lupus.

Other symptoms are similar to those in other auto-immune diseases: flu-like symptoms and skin rashes. The kidneys and liver may become involved in a few cases. The arthritis is treated in the same way as other systemic (ie not joint-specific) forms, while artificial tears and saliva are employed to do what the glands cannot.

Muscular rheumatic conditions

Some doctors are often sceptical about conditions in which the pain seems to be caused in the muscles rather than the joints. It is very difficult to detect this sort of pain clinically – it won't show up on X-rays – so some doctors might claim that it is 'all in the mind'. And, because the joints aren't directly involved, some rheumatologists don't think this sort of thing is their province anyway. They might try to refer a patient to a neurologist or psychiatrist. None of this is good news for the people who have these conditions.

Look up 'fibrositis' or 'polymyalgia rheumatica' (PMR) in a medical dictionary and, if you find anything at all, you will probably see them described as rare. People working in the arthritis field are less convinced.

Fibrositis

Fibrositis, which is caused by the muscles never really relaxing, is probably quite common among people over 50. Constant muscular tension puts strain on the ligaments, causing pain and disturbing sleep. Relaxing the muscles through appropriate exercise, which may also improve posture, can help. So can relaxation techniques.

Polymyalgia rheumatica

As far as symptoms are concerned, polymyalgia rheumatica has much in common with inflammatory arthritis. It is often accompanied by flu-like illness and fatigue, and stiffness is more pronounced in the morning. The disease itself actually affects the muscles. It is rare in people under 50, but is probably more common than often thought in people over this age.

The muscular pain is noticeably different from that experienced after over-exertion or exercise. The inflammation may involve the blood vessels over the skull, resulting in tender temples and perhaps some pain on chewing (called temporal arteritis). Polymyalgia rheumatica will also affect a person's erythrocyte sedimentation rate (ESR), which can be measured by a simple blood test (for more about ESR, see p 24). Certainly, if polymyalgia rheumatica is suspected and the doctor does not offer a blood test, one should be requested.

The condition responds quickly and well to drug treatment, though it may last for a year or two.

Osteoporosis

Osteoporosis is a bone disease rather than a joint disease but is often found in people with arthritis, particularly older people. Bone cells are constantly being replaced, like those in any organ. The process slows with ageing (bone is strongest at between 30 and 40 years of age) and can, if it slows too much, cause the bony tissue to be replaced with fatty tissue and the bones to become thinner and more brittle and fracture more easily – osteoporosis. This can cause particular pain in the spine and hips, and is the most common cause of hip fracture. It is more common in fair-skinned people and among those who are lightly built. The disease affects as many as 1 in 4 post-menopausal women and, in the same age group, 1 in 40 men.

Osteoporosis tends to run in families. The risk of the disease is also increased by:

- lack of exercise;
- early menopause;
- the use of oral steroids or antacids – both of which are used in treating arthritis – over a sustained period;
- low intake of calcium and vitamin D, particularly in childhood;
- certain other diseases such as those of the liver, thyroid or lungs.

These risks are increased by smoking cigarettes and drinking too much alcohol.

In osteoarthritis the bone mass tends to increase, so people with this type of arthritis may be at less risk of osteoporosis. Having said that, this effect may well be offset by the side (unwanted) effects of typical arthritis drugs, as mentioned above. This is certainly the case in rheumatoid arthritis. Here the risk of osteoporosis is also higher because oral steroids can deplete the bones' calcium.

The menopause is an important watershed because the female hormone oestrogen stimulates the production of vitamin D and calcitonin, which help maintain bone mass. Not surprisingly, the risk of osteoporosis increases when production of this hormone stops. Reduced height after the menopause may be an indication of bone weakness.

For post-menopausal women at risk of osteoporosis, hormone replacement therapy (HRT) may be an option. It involves taking oestrogen by mouth, through a skin patch or gel or by means of a small implant beneath the skin. Ideally, HRT should begin before the menopause but the treatment can be started any time after menstruation ceases. HRT slows or may even stop the rate of loss of bone mass but does not replace the lost bony tissue. As with any treatment, there are risks to consider. Some people sleep better and feel more energetic but others feel unnatural. Risks of breast cancer and cancer of the uterus may be increased, but the latter risk may be offset by taking the other female hormone, progesterone, with the oestrogen. It is also worth noting that HRT reduces the risk of heart and lung disease. Other types of osteoporosis treatment such as calcitonin or etidronate drugs may help to rebuild bone, and may be useful if HRT is unsuitable (eg for men).

Some specific exercises can help once the bone mass is reduced but osteoporosis is best prevented at an earlier stage by a healthy diet, particularly in childhood, and through regular weight-bearing exercise, especially in middle age and upwards. Weight-bearing exercise means just that. Swimming, for example, while a great form of exercise is not weight-bearing. Walking is. Exercise is discussed in more detail on page 38.

Because prevention is better than cure, younger people with arthritis, particularly younger women with rheumatoid arthritis, need to be aware of the long-term risks of osteoporosis.

The main problems caused by arthritis

This section gives an overview of some of the types of problems that can be caused by arthritis. Obviously the detail will vary from individual to individual.

The information here needs to be seen in context. Yes, arthritis is serious. Yes, the problems it brings can be major ones. But no, it is not the end of the world. It might just seem like it as you read the next few paragraphs. That's OK. That's how most people with arthritis feel when they are first diagnosed. But, as the rest of this book will demonstrate, the majority of the difficulties can be overcome. Most people with arthritis can lead the lives they want. Some even say that arthritis is one of the best things that ever happened to them because it has taught them so much about themselves.

Pain

For most people with arthritis, the main symptom is pain. In a membership survey by Arthritis Care, 97 per cent of people with arthritis had experienced pain in the previous week. Sometimes the pain is very severe. Often it is continual: in the Arthritis Care survey, over a third were in pain all the time.

As we all know, the physical sensation of pain is bad enough but that is not all it brings. Pain can make it difficult to do everyday things – even turning the pages of this book. It can make movement difficult both for the person with arthritis and for any carer trying to help them to move. To be lifted, even touched, can be excruciating. Pain is mentally as well as physically draining: it can make you tired and erode your self-confidence. Unchecked pain can send anyone into a downward spiral. (More about this in relation to arthritis on page 48.)

The experience of pain and the ability to cope with it vary from individual to individual. The only person who really knows how bad the pain is is the person feeling it. It is an area where you simply

15

cannot make judgements based on your own experience, even your own experience of arthritis.

Lack of mobility

Both damaged joints and painful joints can be difficult to move. People with arthritis in the lower body, including the hips and knees, may well have difficulty with walking and sitting. Some may use a wheelchair. People with the disease in the upper body, particularly the hands and fingers, will have problems with many of the ordinary tasks of day-to-day living. Nearly all of these will be the sort of thing most of us take for granted, so you need to think hard about what the person you are caring for may have trouble with. Undoing a jar, turning a key, switching on an appliance, turning a tap on or off – the list is longer than you think. The little things add up, so it can become difficult to wash or dress oneself. Outside, even if it is possible to get down the steps from the house, is it feasible to get to the nearest shop?

Fatigue

Dealing on a daily basis with pain and lack of mobility can be exhausting. With inflammatory types of arthritis, the disease itself can also be very tiring. There may be flu-like and feverish symptoms, which can be very severe. Imagine the worst flu you've ever had and then some. Many people with arthritis will joke that it affects the brain. It doesn't, of course, but pain and tiredness do have an impact on memory and concentration.

What arthritis will *not* affect is anyone's capacity to make decisions. In fact, it can be argued that disability is good for the brain because disabled people become experts at detailed thinking and coming up with solutions to problems.

What is disability?

More people are disabled by arthritis than by any other medical condition. But what images spring to mind when you think about disabled people?

There are usually two main ones – victim or hero. The media particularly like the heroes – people who have triumphed over their disability and achieved despite it. Examples involving people with arthritis include the woman who climbed Everest, the boy who got a degree, the girl who does ballet and the man who ran a marathon. They think these stories sell newspapers. Most are patronising, and they all dwell on the strangeness of difference. Meanwhile, the charities often emphasise the victim image in order, they believe, to obtain people's sympathy and donations.

It's no wonder that the general public are so scared of X disease or Y impairment. They know they are not heroes so they are terrified of becoming victims. Of course, most people with disabilities aren't heroes or victims at all, they are just ordinary people who happen to have X or Y.

The problem is that these images put a barrier between people with a disability and people without. Think about disability for a moment. Most people, including most doctors, see disability as a medical problem. Disabled people have a disease that needs to be cured. But *is* the disease the real issue? Imagine the following scenario. You want to go to the cinema but you can't because the cinema has steps outside, which you cannot get up because of the arthritis in your knees. What is really stopping you getting into the cinema – the arthritis or the steps? It is a lot easier, quicker and cheaper to build a ramp than to find a cure for arthritis. Looked at this way, disability becomes a social problem. It is society that disables through the barriers – real and metaphorical – that it places in the way of disabled people. Remove the barriers – whether they are a flight of stairs or individuals' prejudices – and you remove the disability. This is sometimes referred to as the social model of disability. It is a really useful way to begin to see beyond the problems to the solutions.

Of course, it is important to think carefully about the medical aspects of arthritis and to explore any new treatments or ideas but don't become obsessed with finding a cure. Even when cures for arthritis emerge – and it won't be in our lifetimes – they will not help the vast majority of people who have the disease today and certainly not those whose disease is so advanced that they have care needs.

Society, in contrast to damaged joints, can change and is changing. The Disability Discrimination Act 1995 makes it illegal to discriminate against disabled people in employment, in providing goods and services, and in selling or letting land or property. However, the Act – and this is why it is far from perfect – does allow discrimination if the provider has a justifiable reason for giving less favourable treatment. The Government is setting up a Disability Rights Commission to help disabled people secure their rights under the Act and to advise about any 'appropriate subsequent law'. As a carer you can really help disabled people by joining their push towards equality.

What is it like to have arthritis?

Meet two people with arthritis who have different degrees of care needs: Joy and Sarah.

Joy's story

There is no typical arthritis story but Joy's raises many of the issues that people with arthritis consider important. She is in her fifties and has osteoarthritis, the most common form of the disease.

Joy

'After arthritis was diagnosed, I was put on the anti-inflammatory drug ibuprofen and I was on it for 15 years. Eventually I said to my doctor that I was worried my stomach would go. She said, "If your stomach was going to go, it would have gone years ago." Then I got a peptic ulcer. I went back to the doctor and challenged her. She said, "What was the point of my alarming you?"

'I know now that ulcers are a not uncommon side effect of anti-inflammatory drugs, but if anything the ulcer has been worse in some ways than the arthritis. It was the ulcer that caused my retirement from work.

'When I first had arthritis, it was difficult for everybody I know. People wanted to do too much. Now family and friends know there isn't anything I can't do – it just takes time. Initially, I was terribly ungracious but the truth is: if you don't know how to handle your arthritis, how can you expect other people to know how to handle it?

'I have been very proud over the years. I didn't want to seem different. Now it doesn't bother me. Sometimes I used a wheelchair at work. It made me self-sufficient. Without it, I couldn't have done half of what I did; I wouldn't have been able to carry anything. Also, I still had enough energy left when I got home to do my housework and voluntary work. But work colleagues found it hard to come to terms with. They would see me walking one day and using a wheelchair the next. They thought I should always be the same or else I was exaggerating on the bad days. They didn't understand that that's how arthritis is. I've stopped trying to justify using the wheelchair some times and not others. If people can't accept me as I am, forget it.

'Arthritis has made me a much better person. I can now appreciate other people's problems much more. Before I had arthritis I used to think that I was sympathetic and understanding, but I didn't really understand; I had no idea. I'm sorry I had to have it but it has enhanced my life – I have much more empathy.'

From Getting a Grip: Self-help for arthritis *by Jim Pollard; Headline 1996*

Sarah's story

Many people with arthritis are carers too. Sarah has arthritis and her husband Peter has a heart condition.

Sarah

'I have osteoarthritis but my husband has had a number of heart attacks so we care for each other. He helps me dress and we try do the housework between us. But he's one of these blokes who has to do it all at once. He can't do a little at a time. That worries me. He can move around more than me but, because his heart is involved, his condition is potentially more life-threatening.

'I'd like a home help but it would be difficult. My husband wouldn't let me have one when it was first offered after my knee operation. Even now I don't think he'd like it. I think he does more than he should and that makes me feel guilty, as I think I should be doing more. I did much more after his last heart attack but I really paid for it. What's more, people see me walking around and don't realise the problems I have. For example, we have a disabled parking space but the neighbours keep using it. They see me walking and so they resent my having a special space.

'They don't know all the problems I had with my operation. I had to have it done twice. Now the surgeons would like to operate on my spine but I don't want them to. I go to a pain clinic because I've been on pain-killers so long I'm beginning to have problems with my stomach. I found a TNS machine that could help but then I developed an allergic reaction to the pads.

'Hydrotherapy helps. The other thing that helps is reducing stress. I felt much better when we went on holiday. But avoiding stress is very hard. As well as Peter's heart, we've had a few problems with our children which hasn't helped the arthritis – it's definitely worse when I feel stressed. I can get depressed, too. With hindsight I think a lot of the bouts of depression that I've had can be put down to arthritis and vice versa. I often wonder exactly how the two are related.

'But there is one advantage in us both having problems. I think it helps us to understand each other's difficulties more.'

For more *i*nformation

ℹ️ Much of the information in this section is amplified in my book *Getting a Grip – Self-help for arthritis and rheumatism* (published by Headline; now out of print but you may be able to get a copy through your local library).

ℹ️ More detailed information on the medical aspects of arthritis can be found in the leaflets published by the Arthritis Research Campaign and in Arthritis Care's booklet *What Is Arthritis?*

ℹ️ *Talk About Pain*, a booklet published by Arthritis Care.

2 How is arthritis treated?

This chapter outlines the main tests that may be carried out to diagnose arthritis. It then looks at the sorts of things a person with arthritis needs to think about when managing their disease. The information will be useful to any carer who wants to understand more about how the disease is treated. It includes treatments that doctors will suggest, such as drugs, but many you will need to seek out for yourself, such as complementary therapies and self-help groups. It should give you a good idea of the sort of people someone with arthritis might want to talk to.

Mei-Lee

'I went to see my GP because, although not exactly in pain, I was very aware of my knees. She tested the movement in my legs and said she could hear a grating sound at my knees, so it might well be osteoarthritis. She sent me to the local hospital for X-rays, and they confirmed her diagnosis.'

Diagnosing arthritis

Osteoarthritis is usually diagnosed readily without X-rays or blood tests. However, if the symptoms are complex, pretty soon the GP should do some blood tests and arrange for an X-ray. Tests are used in four ways:

- to assist in diagnosis;
- to assess the severity of a disease;
- to assess the effects of a treatment;
- to check for side effects.

Which tests are appropriate will depend on the individual and the type of arthritis. In many larger practices these may be done on the premises by a practice nurse; smaller ones will refer the person to the local hospital.

X-rays will be taken of the painful joints, and possibly also of adjacent joints and of the feet if rheumatoid arthritis is suspected. The feet are X-rayed because the physical changes caused by rheumatoid arthritis often appear there first. Other diagnostic techniques include ultrasound scanning, magnetic resonance imaging (MRI) and bone densitometry (bone density) scans. All these enable the doctor to get an idea of the appearance and state of the bones and joints. They won't show pain – patients need to tell doctors about this themselves.

Blood tests

The study of the blood is called haematology, and blood tests are done in the haematology department. The tests typically used in arthritis are as follows.

Red cell count Red cells contain haemoglobin, which carries oxygen into and carbon dioxide out of the body via the lungs. A low haemoglobin level (anaemia) may indicate a deficiency in iron or vitamins or, in rheumatoid arthritis, disease activity. In this last case, monitoring haemoglobin levels helps monitor the disease:

worsening anaemia may suggest a complication. People taking the more powerful anti-arthritis drugs are regularly screened because on rare occasions these drugs may reduce the bone marrow cells that form blood.

The erythrocyte sedimentation rate (ESR) test This test measures the speed at which red blood cells settle under gravity. Inflammation increases the rate of settlement: the quicker the rate, the higher the ESR. A high ESR may, alongside other factors, show that the patient's arthritis is becoming more active and causing more inflammation. On the other hand, it might indicate that there is some other inflammation, and the doctor will have to use their judgement as well as the test results.

The CRP test This monitors levels of the C-reactive protein (CRP) in the blood. As with the ESR, a high level suggests more inflammation due to arthritis. It is rather more specific than the ESR.

White cell count White cells help defend the body against foreign invaders. A rise in their numbers indicates an infection or perhaps, because of the increased auto-immune activity involved, conditions such as rheumatoid arthritis or lupus. The doctor can learn more from closer examination of the three types of white cells (polymorphs, macrophages and lymphocytes) – a rise in one, perhaps, and not the others. A reduced lymphocyte count, for example, is typical of lupus. Drugs can also reduce the number of white cells and this is why patients taking certain stronger drugs need to have a monthly blood test.

Platelet count Platelets are essential for blood-clotting. They are measured because, like white cells, they can be reduced by certain drugs.

Rheumatoid factor At least 70 per cent of people with rheumatoid arthritis have an unusual protein – called rheumatoid factor – in their blood. (People with rheumatoid factor are sometimes termed sero-positive.) It is not the cause of the disease, and many people with the rheumatoid factor never get rheumatoid arthritis. On the other hand, people who get rheumatoid arthritis often develop the rheumatoid factor over time. There is some evidence that people with a particularly high rheumatoid factor develop a more severe disease. The mystery is: why do over three-quarters of people with rheumatoid factor *not* have the condition?

Patient power

You might think that 'patient power' is just another slogan, but it really does work and at absolutely no cost to anyone. Being in control of the management of their arthritis can make people feel better.

David

'One thing I've learned is that there is no one treatment for arthritis. It's not just about taking the drugs – you need to do several things and get a balance between, say, rest and exercise or keeping busy and being relaxed. Nobody will tell you what is best for you; you need to find out for yourself. Make sure your doctors know about the things you're trying, obviously, but don't expect them to know all the answers.'

Well worth considering by anyone with arthritis are courses in self-management and in personal development. Arthritis Care run some excellent ones. These give people with arthritis the opportunity to get together with others with the disease and with trainers who also have arthritis, to share experiences, learn from each other and boost self-esteem. Some courses deal with specific issues such as finding and keeping a job.

Anyone who is unsure about such a course is in good company. 'I didn't fancy it all,' says Jean Thompson who has rheumatoid arthritis. 'For thirty years I'd deliberately not had contact with anyone else with arthritis.' Now she's the manager of Arthritis Care's 'Challenging Arthritis' programme.

Jean

'I was very sceptical at the start of my course but after three weeks I realised that bringing together people who had nothing in common on the surface other than their arthritis could really work. I learned so much. I realised that my pattern of operating had been damaging my health. I used to have a flare every three years but now I've gone six years without one through listening more to my body. When it's a bad day I don't take anything on. 'Challenging Arthritis' cemented this in me. I began a calmer life. *[She has since tutored on nine such courses.]* People are empowered by the programme to look after themselves. They meet as equals. The ethos is sharing. Everybody has the opportunity to stand back and reflect. Everybody has the opportunity to be successful. I used to do a lot of negative thinking – not now.'

People are equally enthusiastic about personal development courses.

Joyce

'I'm a lot more positive now. I'd recommend a personal development course to anyone. You've got nothing to lose and everything to gain. You just need to be prepared to take a hard look at yourself, which can be difficult.'

For more *i*nformation

For information about courses in self-management and personal development, contact the training team at Arthritis Care (address on p 148).

Drug treatments

A key way of controlling arthritis is by medication. Most people with the condition will be taking prescribed drugs (medicines), often more than one and often over a prolonged period. It is important that the person with the disease knows what they are taking and why. As a carer you can help them to do this – by making sure the doctor explains everything fully, for example – but the organisation and maintenance of their drug regimen is not, in most cases, something that it is helpful for you to take over. However, you can both read the information on the drug packaging. If either of you has any questions, ask the pharmacist to explain. This section includes basic information on the main types of drugs used to treat arthritis. It is not for self-prescription but should enable you and the person you are caring for to quiz the doctor more effectively.

According to the Department of Health, over 500 million prescriptions were written by doctors in the UK in 1997, and the Arthritis Research Campaign estimate that about 26 million of them were to treat arthritis. Arthritis Care's membership survey in the early 1990s suggests that four out of five people with arthritis are taking prescribed drugs.

All drugs used in the UK must be licensed by the Medicines Control Agency. They check that research and trials have been conducted to a sufficient standard and indicate how the product may be used. There are three categories:

- *prescription-only drugs*, which are prescribed by a doctor or dentist and supplied by a pharmacist;
- *pharmacy medicines*, or 'over-the counter' medicines, which can be bought without a prescription but only in a pharmacist/chemist shop (eg stronger pain-killers);
- *general sales list (GSL) drugs*, which can be bought pretty much anywhere, including supermarkets.

The last group includes paracetamol, ibuprofen and aspirin. Buying these drugs by their generic (chemical) names is cheaper than

27

buying them by their more familiar brand names (such as Panadol, Nurofen or Anadin).

All drugs, even those only on the general sales list, can have side effects. Side effects are a fact of life. All drugs, from coffee to cocaine, have them. Many will be pretty harmless but some may be dangerous. Make sure that the person with arthritis knows what these risks are and what to look out for. It is the doctor's responsibility to make sure the patient understands. It is the patient's responsibility to report a possible side effect as soon as possible.

In arthritis treatment, drugs can do three things:

- relieve pain;
- reduce inflammation;
- help suppress disease activity.

Doing these things can cause side effects, and other drugs may be prescribed to offset them. It is important *always* to follow the instructions given for each drug, and never to exceed the stated dose.

Analgesics

Analgesics reduce pain. Some of these pain-killers can be bought over the counter (such as paracetamol) whereas the harder-hitting versions, called narcotics, are available only on prescription. Alcohol should be avoided with all analgesics.

Paracetamol is non-narcotic: it works outside the brain. Side effects are unusual, *provided* – and this is important – the stated dose is not exceeded. An overdose can damage the liver, and kill.

Narcotics mimic the action of the body's natural pain-killers (called endorphins) and block the transmission of pain within the brain. They can cause sickness, fatigue or constipation, and may make breathing difficult. Long-term use produces tolerance, requiring a bigger dose to get the same effect – which obviously increases the risk of any side effects. Narcotics include morphine, buprenorphine, codeine, diamorphine, dihydrocodeine and pethidine.

You may also encounter 'combination' analgesics that combine a narcotic and a non-narcotic. Co-codamol, for example, contains paracetamol and codeine. Again, it is important to ensure that the maximum dose of paracetamol is not exceeded – especially if ordinary paracetamol is being taken as well (whether on its own or in, for example, Lem-Sip).

Some drugs prescribed as analgesics are actually anti-inflammatory drugs; for example, aspirin and ibuprofen used in lower doses. This type of drug is discussed in the next section.

Anti-inflammatory drugs

Possibly as many as 20 million prescriptions for non-steroidal anti-inflammatory drugs (NSAIDs) are written every year. They are by far the most commonly prescribed anti-arthritis drug. The first NSAID was the one drug everybody has heard of – aspirin.

There are many, many NSAIDs and the mixture of all the names – both generic (chemical) names and brand names – can send the head spinning quicker than any drug. The advantage is that there are plenty more to choose from if a particular NSAID does not work or produces unacceptable side effects.

NSAIDs have an analgesic (pain-killing) effect but their main use in arthritis is to reduce inflammation. Because of the way they work – they block the production of prostaglandins, a 'chemical messenger' in the immune system that maintains inflammation – NSAIDs usually need to be taken for some time (as long as four weeks in some cases) before there is enough in the bloodstream to have any effect. Moreover, because the body produces prostaglandins all the time, the benefits of NSAIDs are short-lived once they are stopped.

But the immune system is complex. Prostaglandins have a role in all inflammation. For example, they are involved in constantly repairing minor damage to the stomach wall or the gut. Inhibiting the work of prostaglandins in the body can thus result in gastrointestinal problems, and these are frequent with long-term use of NSAIDs. In some cases, ulcers can be severe – if, for example, they form near an artery and cause bleeding. This can need prompt hospital treatment, although fatalities from ulcers are rare.

29

The kindest NSAID on the stomach seems to be ibuprofen, but, even though it can be bought without a prescription, it should not be taken without telling the doctor. Moderately safe NSAIDs include diclofenac, naproxen and indometacin. A new generation of drugs in development (called COX-2) are more targeted in their effects on prostaglandins, and so are better for the stomach. They might gradually replace NSAIDs over the next few years.

Because of the possible risk to the stomach or lining of the intestine, people with arthritis are often prescribed an anti-ulcer drug to be taken with their NSAID. Some products combine an NSAID with an anti-ulcer drug in a single tablet.

Other risks from long-term use of NSAIDs include anaemia (which should be checked for by regular blood tests) and, more rarely, liver, kidney and skin reactions. NSAIDs should be avoided by people with asthma and by pregnant women in their first three months of pregnancy or near delivery.

Many pain-relief creams contain NSAIDs. This is obviously a safer way to take a drug but it is not effective in all cases.

Disease-modifying anti-rheumatic drugs (DMARDs)

Until recently the sensible but cautious approach taken by doctors to treat inflammatory arthritis would begin with pain-killers, then NSAIDs, moving on to DMARDs if necessary, and steroids for flare-ups. A newer approach adopted by most rheumatologists is to act as soon as possible to prevent inflammatory systems getting established in the patient's body. Because pain-killers and NSAIDs do not affect this, they prescribe DMARDs as soon as the diagnosis of arthritis is confirmed. The drug 'of choice' now is methotrexate (see p 31), which is effective and well tolerated by many people. (Most people give up on gold (see p 31) after a few years, but they can stay on low-dose methotrexate.) Of course, all drugs have unwanted effects, but so does untreated disease, so it is important for the patient and doctor to discuss the options and choose the right balance for the individual concerned.

The main DMARDs are:

- **immuno-suppressors** (see below);
- **EC-sulfasalazine** – taken with water after food (plenty of water should be drunk to prevent any kidney reaction). 'EC' means enteric-coated – a special coating that allows the tablet to pass through the stomach before releasing its contents.
- **gold injections** – usually given in the buttock;
- **oral gold** – better tolerated than gold injections but less effective;
- **penicillamine** – taken one hour before or after food. Iron tablets should not be taken within an hour and a half of taking penicillamine;

All DMARDs are potent drugs. Many can reduce the production of red or white blood cells, so regular blood tests are required to monitor the situation. Urine tests are also used with gold and penicillamine because of the possibility of kidney damage. (Sulfasalazine may turn the urine orange but this is harmless.)

People taking penicillamine often report a loss of the sense of taste but it tends to return within six weeks or so regardless of whether or not they are still taking the drug. Tinnitus (a ringing in the ears) has been reported with sulfasalazine. Other DMARD side effects include nausea, diarrhoea, skin rashes and mouth ulcers.

Immuno-suppressors

Immuno-suppressors are slow-acting drugs that damp down the immune system rather than tackling pain or inflammation directly. NSAIDs or analgesics will probably be prescribed as well. Immuno-suppressors might also be used in order to keep the dose of steroids as low as possible (see p 34).

Methotrexate (brand names: Emtexate or Maxtrex) was originally developed for the treatment of leukaemia, and **cyclophosphamide** (brand name: Endoxana) was developed initially to slow the growth of cancer cells. At lower doses they can be used to counter the rapid cell growth that occurs when inflammatory processes start up in diseases such as rheumatoid arthritis or lupus.

Methotrexate is generally taken after the evening meal. It may be taken once a week or daily. The daily dose begins low (around 2.5mg) and rises to 7.5–20mg. Folic acid may be prescribed if the person feels sick after taking the medicine. Methotrexate can cause skin rashes, ulcers or soreness in the mouth, vomiting and diarrhoea. It can also react with alcohol, making drinking inadvisable. In a few people it may cause increasing breathlessness, so the drug must be stopped to prevent damage to the lungs.

Cyclophosphamide is usually taken as a tablet in the morning with food, although in hospital it may be given intravenously. It can cause haemorrhagic cystitis, which makes passing water painful and blood appears in the urine. Drinking lots of water can minimise this risk. Cyclophosphamide can also cause hair loss and irregular menstrual periods.

Both methotrexate and cyclophosphamide can affect fertility. Women should stop taking the drug several months before trying to conceive. Men should stop methotrexate six months before trying, and cyclophosphamide is best avoided altogether.

Other immuno-suppressors such as **cyclosporin A** (Sandimmun) and **azathioprine** (Azamune or Imuran) were first produced to prevent rejection in people who had received an organ transplant. Azathioprine is taken once or twice a day after food in doses up to 2.5mg per kilo of body weight.

Because they act on the immune system, immuno-suppressors can reduce resistance to infectious disease. Like other DMARDs, they can also reduce red cell production and, again, blood tests should be done regularly to monitor the situation.

Anti-malarial drugs

Drugs such as **hydroxychloroquine** (brand name: Plaquenil) and **chloroquine** (brand name: Avloclor), which were originally developed for the treatment of malaria, are often used in the treatment of lupus and sometimes for rheumatoid arthritis. They are usually taken with food once or twice daily. The safe dose depends on the individual's body weight so it is important to monitor any changes here.

The major side effect is the possibility of damage to the retina of the eye. For this reason regular eye tests should be given. Other side effects include stomach upsets, disturbed sleep, skin rashes, dizziness and headaches.

Steroids

Steroids have an important part to play in the body. Produced naturally by the adrenal glands, these chemical messengers travel round in the blood doing all sorts of useful jobs. One particular group, **corticosteroids**, are involved in the metabolism (breaking down) of food and affect the balance of water and salt in the body. However, it is because they are also involved in regulating inflammation and the immune system that they can be used to treat inflammatory diseases. Strictly speaking, when people talk about the steroids used in the treatment of arthritis, they actually mean corticosteroids. Corticosteroids are nothing like anabolic steroids used, often illegally, by some athletes and body-builders.

A synthetic version of corticosteroid is used in rather higher doses than the body would produce naturally. It can be injected directly into the inflamed joint or used as a tablet to combat more general inflammation and to suppress the immune system.

Injections

Giving an injection concentrates the steroid in the crucial area, reducing the chances of the side effects that can occur with a tablet. First, the skin over the joint is cleaned with cotton wool and alcohol and, in some cases, fluid is removed from the joint using a syringe. Then a small dose of steroid and local anaesthetic is injected. The joint should be rested for a day or so, however good it might feel! At the site of the injection there may be a thinning in the fat beneath the skin and a loss of skin colour.

Tablets

Prednisolone is the main steroid taken by mouth (there are others that are injected) but is available in a number of brand names (eg

Deltacortril Enteric, Precortisyl, Prednesol, Sintisone). It is usually taken as one tablet in the morning after food. It is a powerful anti-inflammatory. However, this power is difficult to target – corticosteroids go in all guns blazing – so side effects can be a big problem. Steroids are generally used while waiting for other treatments (DMARDS) to kick in, or during a flare-up or when there are complications in the disease such as the involvement of major organs or the possibility of vasculitis (inflamed blood vessels).

Oral steroids take over from the body's natural source of corticosteroids, the adrenal glands, so the body quickly becomes dependent on the tablets. This means that oral steroids should never be stopped suddenly. The body needs to be weaned off them to allow the adrenal glands to start doing their job again. Anyone taking steroids should carry a card (which the doctor should provide) or wear a medical information bracelet so that the dose can be continued in the event of an accident.

Side effects

The side effects from taking steroids continuously can be serious, so a patient should consider them carefully and discuss them with their doctor before embarking on a steroid programme. Equally, however, they need to be aware of the potential dangers of not treating their disease.

Side effects can include: water retention, causing a bloated feeling; muscle fatigue; and the redistribution of weight from the arms and legs to the face and body. This last coupled with the water retention can cause weight gain. Skin can become thin, bruise easily and become prone to rashes and acne. Calcium loss can lead to thinning of the bones and osteoporosis. People taking steroids can become more prone to illness and infection, because of the effect on the immune system. High doses may also affect blood pressure, mood and sleep. In extreme cases, steroids may cause heart failure.

For all these reasons, doses should be kept as low as possible, so steroids are often used with DMARDs. It is generally considered that major side effects are unlikely to occur at doses below 7.5mg per day. At this level the adrenal glands still have to do some work of their own. Sometimes steroids might be prescribed to be taken every other day, rather than every day.

High-dose steroids are avoided nowadays. However, sometimes it is necessary to use a high dose for a few weeks and then gradually reduce it. The doctor will always give high priority to reducing potentially damaging inflammation.

New drugs

Several new arthritis drugs are expected to become available in 2000, according to *Arthritis News*.

As well as the COX-2 inhibitors mentioned on page 30, which are kinder to the stomach than existing NSAIDs, there is an important new generation of drugs to treat rheumatoid arthritis. These 'biological response modifiers' are genetically engineered to block the action of tumour necrosis factor (TNF), which plays a key role in the inflammation of rheumatoid arthritis. There are also new drugs for osteoarthritis, containing synthetic hyaluronic acid, which helps shock absorption and lubrication in the joints.

A concern of arthritis organisations is that these drugs are expensive, which might lead to problems with what is called 'post-code rationing' whereby some hospitals provide the drugs while others cannot afford to do so.

Drug names to ask your doctor about include:

- for osteoarthritis – hyaluronate (brand name: Hyalgan) and hylan G-F 20 (Synvisc);
- for rheumatoid arthritis – infliximab (brand name: Remicade), etanercept (Enbrel) and leflunomide (Arava);
- COX-2 inhibitors – celecoxib (Celebrex) and rofecoxib (Vioxx).

How to get the best out of drugs

When the doctor prescribes drugs for you or the person you are caring for, make sure you know exactly what they are. It can take time to find the right drug and the right dosage. Knowing exactly what is being taken helps you to assess the effects.

Ask the doctor:

- What is the drug called? (Both the brand name and the generic name.)
- How many tablets should be taken and how often? Before or after eating? At bedtime? What if a dose is missed?
- What does it do? Is it a pain-killer (analgesic), an anti-inflammatory, a disease modifier?
- What specific benefits should it bring?
- How quickly will it work? (Some drugs work more quickly than others.)
- How strong is it? (In milligrams.)
- What are the possible side effects? Is there anything that can be done to prevent them? What should be done if it seems that the person may be experiencing them?
- Should anything be avoided while taking the drug? Alcohol? Driving? Operating machines?

With certain drugs, such as steroids where it is important that the course of treatment is not interrupted, patients are given an information card which should be carried at all times. With others, such as gold, a record card is provided, to be filled in after every treatment and blood and urine test.

Something that is not always stressed enough in the doctor's surgery is the importance of taking the drugs at the right time and in the right quantity. People use all sorts of methods to remind them: watch alarms, kitchen timers, notes in a diary, good-natured partners and so on. You can even buy a beeping pill box. For best results, drugs should be taken according to the clock and the doctor's instructions, not according to how much pain is felt. Lurching from one extreme to the other makes it harder to assess the effectiveness of the medication and can be very disruptive to everyday life.

It helps the doctor to prescribe the right medication if the patient is blunt about how they feel. Being brave or uncomplaining may lead to the wrong drug or a dose that is too low. Too little of a pain-killer is more likely to lead to dependence than too much, because the body notices the difference it makes far more. And no one should ever feel guilty if what is first prescribed doesn't work. Doctors usually have a system to work through, starting with the most commonly effective drug and dose, and then trying others according to the individual's responses.

Patients should be frank with their doctor about side effects. With NSAIDs, for example, a number of strategies can be employed to reduce stomach pain: spreading the dose (more frequent doses of weaker tablets); changing the time at which the dose is taken (eg after eating when the stomach lining is coated); trying a coated tablet (which will pass through the stomach before releasing its contents); or taking an antacid with the drug. This advice also applies to any over-the-counter aspirin.

Prescriptions can be expensive for most patients between the ages of 18 and 60. At the time of writing, they cost £5.90 an item and the charge tends to rise every year. Despite lobbying by patients' organisations, a person with arthritis does not qualify for free prescriptions as do some people with other long-term medical conditions (eg diabetes). However, anyone who has to pay for a lot of prescribed drugs might find a prepaid season ticket helpful. These last for four or twelve months, and holders need pay no more for the NHS prescriptions for the duration of the season ticket. The NHS say that you will benefit if you need over five items in four months or more than 14 items in 12 months. Apply using the FP95 form (EP95 in Scotland), available in the post office.

When buying over-the-counter drugs such as aspirin, ibuprofen or paracetamol, it is cheaper to ask for them by these generic names rather than choose one of the brand names.

For more *i*nformation

ⓘ More information about arthritis drugs can be found in Arthritis Care's series of easy-to-read drug sheets, which were put together with a panel of distinguished health professionals, including leading rheumatologists.

ⓘ *Know Your Medicines* by Pat Blair, published by Age Concern Books.

37

Exercise and leisure activities

The facts about exercise are simple: get enough and you'll feel better, have more energy, be able to do more and might even live longer. People with arthritis need exercise as much as anybody else but must choose more carefully the forms it takes. The fatigue associated with certain types of arthritis and the loss of bone mass in osteoporosis can make a difference to what is appropriate.

Sarah

'We both try to keep active – Peter plays bowls. It's important to keep your mind active as much as anything else. I visit a nursing home and take some of the residents to church or play the organ. It helps me forget my own problems.'

Leisure activities such as sport and gardening can be continued, even if they may need a bit of modification. For example, Disability Sport England (address on p 153) promotes sport for people with disabilities from local to national level. Sport England (address on p 159) encourages sports governing bodies to cater for older people, and provides information on leadership and the addresses of regional sports councils, which will have more local information. Gardeners with disabilities or special needs can obtain advice and information from Thrive (address on p 159). RADAR publishes information giving details of accessibility to, for example, places of interest. Some national organisations, such as the National Trust and English Heritage (addresses on pp 157 and 154), publish guides for visitors with disabilities.

People with arthritis enjoy additional benefits from exercising. It protects against joint damage, keeps joints and muscles working, and helps to prevent disability. Unexercised joints can lose muscle strength, becoming painful and unstable, and cartilage deteriorates faster. So rather than resting arthritic joints, it is even more important to exercise them. Someone with osteoarthritis will not do any damage through exercise, even if it causes some pain. Exercise also helps keep bones strong, which can protect against osteoporosis. Moreover, people who are confident on their feet are less likely to have accidents.

Age is no barrier. Studies show that men and women aged 65 and over can improve their strength, stamina and suppleness considerably within a few weeks of beginning a supervised exercise programme. Most forms of exercise can be done with a friend or partner – for example, walking, dancing or taking part in a class – which will make it an enjoyable activity rather than a boring chore.

There are three types of exercise – stretching, strengthening and endurance exercise. A good programme will include all three, and will take into account the type and severity of the arthritis and the individual's general level of fitness. Sports and health centres often have staff who are qualified to give advice, but people with arthritis should probably consult their GP or physiotherapist before beginning any new exercise programme.

Stretching exercise

Stretching or range of movement (ROM) exercise is the most important for people with arthritis. It involves taking your joints through their full range of movement and then just easing them a little further. This is the sort of exercise people do when warming up for sport; it is excellent for maintaining a joint's mobility and over time may well improve it. Stretching exercises can even be performed on inflamed joints.

Joy

'Exercise is vitally important but so is rest. The difficult bit is the balance. Too much rest and you get stiff; too much exercise and you're in pain. I relax in my garden. If I'm up-tight I just disappear out there.

I don't do much – just a bit of dead-heading or something – but afterwards I'm a different person. I do my stretching exercises anywhere – watching TV, even sitting in the car in traffic jams (I get some funny looks!).'

From Getting a Grip: Self-help for arthritis *by Jim Pollard; Headline 1996*

Strengthening exercise

By tightening and releasing the muscles around a joint, strengthening exercises can help restore its strength and stability. The particular strengthening exercises will depend very much on the location, severity and type of the individual's arthritis. For example, strengthening the quadriceps muscles on the front of the thighs is excellent for arthritis in the knees. Some exercises will be harmful for some people so it is essential to discuss a programme with a health professional. People with painful hips and knees should certainly avoid too many weight-bearing exercises, and heavy weight-lifting is not recommended.

Muscle weakness can be the result of the arthritis itself, of the inactivity it prompts and sometimes of the long-term use of steroid drugs. For this reason some strengthening exercises may be quite difficult at first but they do become easier, especially if done in conjunction with ROM exercise. Strengthening exercise should not be performed on inflamed joints until the pain or swelling has eased, or done only very slowly to minimise the pain.

Endurance exercise

This is the sort of thing we normally think of as exercise – walking, dancing, running, cycling, swimming and so on. When this exercise is 'aerobic' it burns off calories, speeds up the body's metabolism, helps maintain a strong heart and may reduce the harmful type of cholesterol that can clog the arteries. It can also reduce fatigue. To be 'aerobic', it should leave the exerciser slightly breathless (*not* panting) and with an increased pulse (*not* a pounding heart). To be beneficial, it is thought to be important that the exercise is prolonged (20–30 minutes) and regular (at least three times a week). However, recent American studies indicate that a good result can also be obtained by splitting those 20 minutes into, say, five sessions of 4 minutes each. The GP should be consulted before embarking on a new exercise programme.

Forms of exercise popular with people with arthritis include the following:

- **Walking** is a cheap, easy way to get fitter that can be readily incorporated into everyday life. Walking to the shops is much more relaxing than sitting in a traffic jam. People who use a walking stick can usually still benefit from walking unless they experience pain over very short distances.
- **Dancing**, such as ballroom dancing or line dancing, is an excellent, enjoyable way to get exercise that improves mobility and balance.
- **Swimming** is great all-round exercise, stretching and strengthening muscles as well as getting the heart going. The particular benefit of exercising in water is that it supports the body weight, enabling more exercise to be done. The Arthritis Research Campaign say that, for people with rheumatoid arthritis, learning to swim could be one of the best investments they make in their future.
- **Hydrotherapy** is a common treatment for arthritis. The water is generally warmer than in the swimming pool, and exercise is under medical supervision. Ask the GP about local hydrotherapy facilities. Also look out for water-based exercise classes such as aquarobics – aerobics in the pool – or flotation aerobics. People with arthritis attending such classes should avoid straining to reach a position and must make sure that the teacher knows of their condition, as some movements may be inappropriate.
- **Cycling** It's amazing how much modern cycles can be adapted to suit the individual's needs, while static exercise bikes are available for those who don't fancy the road. It is easy to prevent

boredom while using an exercise bike by reading a book, listening to the radio or watching TV at the same time.

■ **Aerobics** There are specific classes aimed at people with disabilities and some have disabled aerobics instructors. High-impact classes where the feet hit the ground vigorously and often are not advised. People with arthritis will probably want to opt for low- or even no-impact exercise. Again, people with arthritis attending aerobics classes should avoid straining to reach a position and must make sure that the teacher knows of their condition, as some movements may be inappropriate.

■ **Sports** Golf, martial arts and t'ai chi, tennis and many other sports are enjoyed by people with arthritis. As always, consult your doctor before embarking on new activities.

Everyday activities, including vacuuming, dusting and cleaning the windows, also stretch the muscles, strengthen them and burn off calories. Approaching these activities with the same care and forethought as one would an exercise can help make them safer.

Exercise guidelines

■ Balance exercise with rest and relaxation.

■ Couple exercise with joint care. Avoid using heavy weights or staying in one position for too long. Kneeling and squatting, for example, should be avoided by anyone with knee problems.

■ Follow the two-hour rule – if more pain is felt two hours after exercising than before, less exercise should be done next time.

■ Little and often within a daily routine is best for ROM and for strengthening exercise.

■ It is best to exercise when pain and stiffness and tiredness are least and medication is having its maximum effect.

■ A warm bath or the application of heat (see p 48 for some ideas) before more prolonged exercise may help relax the muscles.

Exercise has real benefits. It adds life to years and years to life.

It can be fun

Lucy

'I call my favourite exercise "toelympics". Sit down, place a matchbox on the floor with the end up and try to pick it up with your bare toes. Not as easy as it sounds. As you become more proficient, try a mock game of noughts and crosses using alternate feet or even with an opponent!'

Especially with other disabled people

Catriona

'There was a real buzz in the room when we had a disabled aerobics instructor. I could see other people having problems keeping in time as well as me. We just smiled at one another and felt glad we weren't the only ones making a fool of ourselves. It didn't matter, though, because we were all having so much fun.'

And age is no barrier

Rita

'I'm in my 70s now but I am a new person, full of energy, free from any pain; and, to crown it all, my fourth hip operation became unnecessary. The muscles in my legs have become really strong and it seems that the hip joint has repaired itself. I can walk without pain – something that was denied me for 20 years. It is an under-statement to say that exercise is good for you.'

Diet

Diet is still probably the most controversial area in the treatment of arthritis. Some people make incredible claims about it; many doctors are still frankly sceptical. What is clear is that no diet will cure arthritis nor will one particular diet 'work' in all types of the disease.

This is not to say that the role of diet isn't important. If we are what we eat, then we might be able to alter what we are by altering what we eat. Any doctor will tell you that it is always a good idea to think about what you eat, and for people with arthritis it's worth thinking about a little more.

Joy

'I've discovered that citric acid [found in citrus fruit such as oranges and lemons, and artificially as flavouring E330] doesn't seem to agree with me so I try to keep that out of my diet. I don't know if it specifically affects my arthritis but I certainly feel better for avoiding it.'

From Getting a Grip: Self-help for arthritis *by Jim Pollard; Headline 1996*

People with arthritis should certainly aim to eat a healthy diet. This is defined by the Health Education Authority as the following:

■ eat a variety of food to get the full range of nutrients;
■ eat plenty of foods rich in starch and fibre;
■ don't eat too much fat (especially saturated fats such as butter, meat fats);
■ don't eat sugary foods too often;
■ look after the vitamins and minerals when preparing your food;
■ keep alcohol consumption within sensible levels;
■ aim to eat the right amount to be a healthy weight.

Eating a balanced diet should mean that mineral or vitamin supplements are unnecessary. However, for some people, including older people and those with disabilities, they may be appropriate. People with arthritis and osteoporosis should discuss their diet with their GP and ask if any supplements might be necessary.

What many people with arthritis want to know is whether there is anything beyond this that could help them. There are two areas worth considering: specialist dietary supplements and dietary manipulation. Neither has been researched in great depth – certainly not to the satisfaction of most doctors – and most of the research that has been done has been on rheumatoid arthritis.

Common dietary supplements

Fish oils

The fatty acids in fish oil may produce less inflammatory chemicals than those from animal fats, suggesting that fish oil may ease joint pain and stiffness in inflammatory disease such as rheumatoid arthritis and lupus. Dr Gail Darlington, author of Arthritis Care's booklet *Diet and Arthritis*, and one of the leading rheumatologists working in this field, has described the research so far as 'promising'. However, fish oil takes three to six months to become effective and it needs to be taken long term despite the fact that long-term safety has yet to be investigated. Nor has the effect of the lower strength doses that you can buy over the counter. What can be said with more certainty is that fish oil is good for your heart. Fish oils are not available on prescription but can be obtained from most pharmacist/chemist shops and health food shops.

Evening primrose oil (EPO)

Evening primrose oil has effects similar to those of fish oils and takes as long to become effective. Long-term effects have also yet to be investigated. Fish oils and evening primrose oil can be taken together. Again, Dr Darlington sees research so far as 'promising'.

New Zealand green-lipped mussel

Extract of the New Zealand green-lipped mussel may have a mild anti-inflammatory effect, although evidence of its value in rheumatoid arthritis is limited.

Selenium

There is some evidence of a relationship between low levels of the trace element selenium and arthritis but it is not clear whether this can be remedied by a supplement. Selenium by mouth may be toxic in large quantities.

Iron

Anaemia in rheumatoid arthritis does not necessarily respond to iron supplements.

Garlic

Fresh garlic (rather than pearls) is good for the heart but its benefit in rheumatoid arthritis is not yet known.

There is no evidence that any of the supplements mentioned above is helpful in osteoarthritis, though this does not mean they are not in some cases. However, the most beneficial dietary treatment for osteoarthritis is to keep weight down (weight loss is discussed on p 47).

Dietary manipulation

Dietary manipulation will work for only some people with rheumatoid arthritis – perhaps 40 per cent at most. It's a difficult process, which must be under a doctor's supervision to prevent the danger of malnutrition. It can also be disruptive to your life and needs a high level of commitment. If it doesn't work after six weeks, it is important to return to medical treatment to prevent joint damage. There are three stages:

- **elimination** – removing pretty much all but a few simple foods from the diet;
- **reintroduction** – if symptoms disappear following elimination, foods are reintroduced one by one to see if they cause the symptoms to return;
- **challenging** – this involves the removal and reintroduction of what seem to be the problem foods to see if they really are the cause of the symptoms.

The challenging phase is particularly important because initial benefits may simply be the result of the natural ups and downs of rheumatoid arthritis or of the body responding to its starvation by producing more of its own corticosteroids or of a placebo response (discussed on p 55).

One form of arthritis in which changing the diet definitely does help is gout. Foods rich in purines (see the list on p 9) raise the level of uric acid in the blood and this is what causes gout. Fasting, however, can also bring on a gout attack.

Weight loss

Roughly four times our body weight goes through the joints in the lower limbs as we move around, so the less weight the less damage this can cause. An overweight person with osteoarthritis in the knees will benefit from losing weight. This may also be true for someone with osteoarthritis of the hips. Losing a few kilos can help reduce pain and disability.

Unfortunately, losing weight and maintaining the weight loss can be hard. Setting small but achievable monthly goals is often worth trying, perhaps enlisting the help of the GP or practice nurse, or joining a reputable slimming group. If necessary, get advice from the GP or a dietician about the foods to avoid and how to make sure that the overall diet is well balanced and nutritious.

For more *i*nformation

Diet and Arthritis by Dr Gail Darlington, published by Arthritis Care.

Pain control

The main symptom of arthritis is pain. Nearly everyone with arthritis experiences it frequently, while more than a third are in constant pain. This is unpleasant enough but pain can set up a vicious cycle of other problems: pain causes fatigue, which causes depression, which causes stress, which causes more pain. Reducing pain can break the cycle.

Pain control is a personal affair. We all need to mix and match to find what works for us, but it may help to talk to other people to find out how they manage their arthritis.

Rebecca

'I now have my own pain management programme. I take the pain-killers I need, visit an osteopath and use heat and massage for pain relief. If walking hurts, I use my wheelchair and now I pay someone to do my housework instead of struggling on in pain. I keep my pain in place, and if something hurts I don't do it. There's nothing noble about suffering.'

From Talk About Pain, *published by Arthritis Care*

Scientists and pain control specialists have developed the idea of the 'pain gate'. This is located in the spinal cord, and closing it can prevent the nerve signals recognised as pain from ever reaching the brain. It can be closed both physically and mentally.

Three of the main ways of closing the pain gate are discussed elsewhere in this book (drugs – see pp 27–37; complementary therapies – see pp 54–66; exercise – see pp 38–42) but there are others, discussed below.

Heat

Warmth messages can block pain messages by beating them to the pain gate. Applying heat also gets the blood flowing. That's why 'rubbing it better' – or a massage or a TNS machine (see below) – can really help. So can a hot bath, a hot towel, an electric blanket, nice thick sheets (eg flannel) or a hot water bottle (wrapped in a towel).

Heated pads may help. Some of these run off the mains, others use batteries or are heated in the microwave and some are operated with a special disc in the pad itself. Some have thermostats and a massage facility. They are available for various parts of the body but be careful: some are very expensive. Make sure that they are approved to BEAB (British) or CE (European) standards.

Cold

Applying cold numbs pain and, during a flare-up of symptoms, can reduce swelling and muscle spasms. Buy cold packs at the pharmacist/chemist shop or make them by wrapping a damp towel round a pack of frozen vegetables or a bag of crushed ice. Never apply ice direct to the skin. Stop when the affected area feels numb.

TNS (transcutaneous nerve stimulation)

Using a TNS machine involves small electrodes that are taped to the skin and gently vibrate. The minute electrical impulses help close the pain gate by providing an alternative stimulus. Make sure that they are approved to BEAB (British) or CE (European) standards. Some people love them; others find them useless. A lot depends on where the pain is.

Note Anyone with a pacemaker should **not** use TNS.

Joy

'I'm only on pain-killers now because of the ulcer. I use a TNS machine which is extremely good but, because I have spinal arthritis, I can't bend my body enough to actually attach it to the affected parts – the daft thing is, of course, that it's particularly difficult on the days I really need it.'

From Getting a Grip: Self-help for arthritis *by Jim Pollard; Headline 1996*

Occupying the mind

Keeping busy prevents the pain messages swarming around unhindered. This is why as full a life as possible really does help arthritis. But activity needs to be balanced with relaxation. To be most beneficial, relaxing should still occupy the mind. People can think about anything they like, provided they enjoy it. It could be what they will be doing in the future or something they did in the past. It may be family and friends or hobbies. Let the imagination roam free. Or they can try this simple relaxation technique:

■ find a pleasant place where you won't be interrupted and there's nothing more than soft music in the background;
■ sit comfortably, with head supported and eyes closed;
■ breathe deeply, feeling your abdomen rise and fall;
■ focus on your breathing;
■ then think about a favourite place or journey – real or imaginary – or simply think calming words like love and peace.

For other, more focused, uses of the mind, explore meditation or hypnosis.

Sleep

A good night's sleep always helps but pain is usually at its worst from around 10pm, making it difficult to drop off. Altering sleep patterns and avoiding stimulants such as alcohol, cigarettes, tea or coffee in the couple of hours before going to bed might help. Or try a warm bath instead. Make sure that the bed is warm and comfortable (most people with arthritis prefer a firmer bed).

Nobody should feel guilty about taking themselves off to bed at times.

Trudi

'On bad days I indulge myself by watching morning TV in my dressing gown by the fire with a mug of tea. Or I might go to bed in the afternoon with a good book and a hot water bottle. This is part of the way I handle my pain.'

From Talk About Pain, *published by Arthritis Care*

Sex

Making love is one of the best ways of closing the pain gate and probably the most enjoyable one to try.

Penny

'When it's shared with the one you love, sex is a great stress buster. Your awareness of pain may lessen because you are enjoying yourself. Enjoying making love with your partner will also boost self-esteem and help you stay in a positive frame of mind when tackling pain. It is very important to cherish and give attention to your body. Making love, gently and at a time appropriate to you, will have a healing effect. Choose positions that are comfortable. Be adventurous and experiment. Tell your partner what feels good. Sex is the best exercise you can get in a horizontal position, but never forget that cosy hugs and kisses are important too.'

From Talk About Pain, *published by Arthritis Care*

Pain clinics

There are now pain clinics throughout the UK, many attached to hospitals. They were set up by anaesthetists and nurses and others to raise awareness of and meet the needs of people with pain. Some but not all are very good for people with arthritis. The NHS information service on 0800 66 55 44 can provide the address of the nearest pain clinic.

51

For more *i*nformation

ⓘ The NHS information service on 0800 66 55 44 can provide the address of the nearest pain clinic, and is also a good first point of contact for finding out about NHS services.

ⓘ *Talk About Pain*, a booklet published by Arthritis Care.

ⓘ *Our Relationships, Our Sexuality*, a booklet published by Arthritis Care.

Counselling

Counselling can certainly help in pain control. Unloading stress and negative emotions can break the pain cycle, which means that some people find that just talking about how they feel can take the pain away.

Seeking counselling is not a sign of not coping – either with arthritis or with the difficulties of caring or with life in general – rather the opposite. It is doing something about the things that are being troublesome.

Arthritis Care provide an excellent telephone counselling service for people with arthritis and their carers. Give them a call on 0808 800 4050. Counsellors may also be available through your GP, or they can be seen privately. Make sure they are registered with the British Association for Counselling. Fees are usually on a sliding scale depending on the person's resources. The advice on pages 56–58 on finding a complementary therapist you are comfortable with applies equally to counsellors.

Self-help groups

Talking with other people who have arthritis or with other carers can ease feelings of isolation, provide valuable information and support, and be a lot of fun. Arthritis Care has 650 branches and local groups across the UK, aimed at people of all ages and from all sections of the community. Here are two happy Arthritis Care members.

Chris

'To be honest, I went along to be nosy and find out what they did. I found myself talking to everyone. It was very beneficial to be with other people in a similar position to myself, all having some form of arthritis. I felt comfortable with everyone. They were all so lovely and friendly that I assumed they'd all been meeting for years but, in fact, it was only the second get-together they'd ever had. The point is everyone understands the pain and frustrations I have felt. We have lots of laughs at these meetings, discussing our individual experiences of life.'

From Talk About Pain, *published by Arthritis Care*

Les

'It's not the individual activities that attract me to the group – the outings, the speakers and so on – although they are fun. It's the opportunity to talk to people who understand exactly what you're talking about without you having to explain the ins and outs of your problems. I find it supportive, informative and I get strength from it.'

There are also charities and support and self-help groups for people with specific types of arthritis. The more general ones are listed in the 'Useful addresses' section at the back of this book; for more specific groups, see Arthritis Care's magazine *Arthritis News* or ask in your local reference library for a directory of self-help groups.

Self-help groups also benefit carers.

Tom

'We've met a lot of interesting people and learned a lot from Arthritis Care. I met an occupational therapist at one meeting, who came round to assess the changes we needed to the house when my wife got arthritis. That sort of practical thing is happening all the time.'

For more *i*nformation

i Arthritis Care (address on p 148) produces useful booklets on most of the topics discussed above, and provides advice and support for people with arthritis and their carers.

i Carers National Organisation has many local groups; contact the head office (address on p 150) for the one nearest you.

Complementary therapy

The term 'complementary therapy' covers a broad range of different treatments – from those generally accepted by the medical establishment such as chiropractic and osteopathy to those with no foundation in Western science at all. Some, like the two just mentioned, require the manipulation of the body. Others call for new skills to be learned, different lifestyles to be adopted or offer potions or pills. Some claim to work by faith alone. None will cure arthritis but they can help. Remember that no complementary treatment can undo joint damage that has already been done. People with arthritis will want to keep their doctors informed of any complementary therapies they are trying.

All the approaches have one thing in common: someone somewhere thinks they have helped them. The one thing that I would say about them, based on my experience and that of many others, is that there is probably one somewhere that can help most of us.

Including carers. The secret is to pick a way through the maze of complementary therapies to find the one(s) that suit the temperament and the bank balance as well as the medical condition.

Many of the complementary therapies listed in this chapter see the world and the human body within it in a different way from conventional medicine; their notions of research and evidence are not the same as those of Western scientists. Much evidence, for example, is anecdotal, based on people's reports of their own experience, rather than experimental. That does not, of itself, mean that these approaches do not work. Only that it is harder to prove. Sometimes the only way is a 'suck it and see' approach. However, if a fair trial doesn't seem to have achieved anything, people should trust their judgement and move on.

Where pretty much all the complementary therapies differ from mainstream medicine is in what they aim to treat. Mainstream medicine treats the disease; complementary therapy treats the whole person, which immediately yields a benefit – the individual and their views are placed at the centre of the process. To someone with arthritis who is used to being treated like dozens of other similar patients with what can be considered a low-priority, long-term, unglamorous, marginalised condition, this will be enormously liberating.

In this person-centred or holistic approach the first session of most therapies is fairly long, perhaps an hour or even more, because the therapist will take a full personal and medical history. NHS doctors, even with the best will in the world, just do not have this sort of time.

Some doctors say that complementary therapy is just placebo – something that does nothing at all but helps a person who has faith in it. Placebos are used in trials to provide comparative data for the drug under scrutiny: half the people in the trial are given a placebo and the other half are given the new drug. Some of those who are given the placebo still get better. This is called the placebo effect, and some doctors dismiss complementary therapies as nothing more than the placebo effect writ large. Perhaps they are right. Who knows? But is that the most important issue? Most people are simply pleased that they have got better. Leave the scientists to worry about how. The placebo effect only serves to emphasise the power of the mind in health and healing.

The down-side of all this is obvious – anyone can claim anything will cure anything, and how are we to know whether they are telling the truth? There is only moderate regulation of the medical and health claims people can make about themselves and their products. For example, some manufacturers blur the line between a food and a drug to maximise the health benefits they can claim for their products and minimise the regulations.

Some therapies have their own internal regulatory mechanisms and may have a list of registered practitioners who have reached certain standards or undergone certain periods of training. Some but not all. Choose a therapist carefully to minimise the chances of falling into the hands of an unscrupulous one.

The following sections mention some of the complementary therapies that are most popular with people with arthritis. Clearly, no one complementary therapy will work for everybody any more than any one medicine will, but, for people with arthritis, few are actually dangerous. Complementary therapies can help carers, too: you don't have to have a medical condition to benefit. Many of the therapies will simply make you feel good. Feelings of stress and difficulty relaxing or sleeping, for example, which are common in carers are also problems that complementary therapies are particularly good at helping you address.

Finding the right therapist

First, choose a therapy. Possible starters, to improve mobility in stiff (but not inflamed) joints, might be chiropractic, osteopathy or yoga. To reduce pain, consider acupuncture or reflexology. For a feel-good pick-me-up, try aromatherapy or massage.

Joy

'I also use aromatherapy. I read about it in a magazine and sent for the oils. My sister, who is a nurse, makes them up for me and other people with arthritis. I rub them into my skin two or three times a day. The effect doesn't last long but it's very soothing and smells lovely.'

From Getting a Grip: Self-help for arthritis *by Jim Pollard; Headline 1996*

Second, approach the regulatory body for a list of local therapists (the Arthritis Care Helpline or the local library can probably help here). Check just what inclusion on the list means. Does it signify certain qualifications or experience, or merely that a membership fee has been paid? For an unregulated therapy, try word of mouth beginning with the most reliable sources such as a GP or another health professional or therapist before trying friends and relatives. Be very wary of the practitioner who approaches you direct, bearing a broad smile and a special introductory offer. A therapist's effectiveness is often in inverse proportion to the claims they make. Beware of somebody promising the Earth. The most likely result is that your therapy will end up costing it.

Third, ask questions. Before committing to anyone, however highly recommended, check them out.

- What exactly do they do?
- How long have they been doing it?
- How did they start?
- What training have they had? Where? For how long?
- What professional bodies do they belong to?

A key question is whether they are insured. Few insurance companies will insure unqualified practitioners. Members of the Institute for Complementary Medicine should be insured through them. No genuine therapist will mind questioning. After all, if theirs is a person-centred approach, it will be important to them that you feel comfortable.

Make sure you can talk to them. Do you understand what they are on about? Incomprehensible mystical mumbo-jumbo is of no use. Ask what their therapy will involve.

■ How long will each session take?
■ How long will the whole programme take?
■ What sort of benefits might you expect to see? When?

It is obviously important to ask how much it will all cost. Embarking on a programme that you cannot afford may create more problems than it solves. Explore these costs with your GP. The range of therapies to which a doctor can refer a patient is increasing all the time. Occasionally, a voluntary organisation may be able to help. Perhaps there are sessions at a local authority leisure centre or other council facility.

Fourth, ensure that it is your choice. Don't be afraid to change your mind before starting or after a few sessions. Again, no genuine therapist will object. Don't be bullied into staying. If the therapist starts using language that suggests you are responsible for any failure or that makes you feel uncomfortable, head for the door. On the other hand, don't give up if results aren't immediate. Discuss your concerns with the therapist.

Fifth, get into it. Once in a consultation or session with a therapist, leave your scepticism behind. Go with what you have chosen to do and enjoy it. That way you maximise your chances of finding something that really helps.

Acupuncture

Acupuncture is recommended by its practitioners for pain relief, stress and sleep problems, and immune problems.

Basic principles Ancient Chinese. Acupuncture sees ill-health as caused by imbalances in a body's energy (yin and yang). These can be corrected by stimulating the flow of healing chi energy at different acupoints on the body depending on the problem.

Methods of treatment Fine needles are inserted in the acupoints. Most people say it is not painful. As with most complementary therapies, the first session is usually a long one. The acupuncturist will be particularly interested in the client's reactions to the opposites of hot and cold, damp and dry, etc, asking what sort of food is preferred, what time of year and so on.

Length of treatment Three to six sessions are usually needed.

Attitudes of medical doctors Many doctors tend to accept that it can work for some people but suggest that, rather than chi energy, it is the body's natural pain-killing endorphins that are stimulated by the needles. It may also increase the body's own release of corticosteroids.

Related therapies Acupressure and Shiatsu use a similar philosophical approach but with finger pressure instead of needles.

Regulatory body British Acupuncture Council (address on p 150).

Aromatherapy

Aromatherapy is recommended by its practitioners for respiratory problems, skin problems, chronic pain and anything in which stress is an element.

Basic principles Ancient Egyptian, Greek, Roman and Arab. Aromatherapy employs the healing properties of distilled oils from aromatic plants, called essential oils.

Methods of treatment It works primarily through the sense of smell but can often be combined with massage. The art, say practitioners, lies in choosing the right blend of oil for the right person at the right time. A good aromatherapy massage can be very relaxing indeed.

Length of treatment When required.

Attitudes of medical doctors Few would advise against it and most would acknowledge the benefits of massage and of stimulating the senses.

Regulatory body None. Look out for qualifications such as the Associate of Tisserand Aromatherapists (ATA) or membership of bodies such as the International Society of Practising Aromatherapists (ISPA) or the International Federation of Aromatherapists (IFA).

Chiropractic

Chiropractic is recommended by its practitioners for anything to do with the joints and muscles, including neck and back pain, headaches and tension.

Basic principles Developed by Canadian Daniel David Palmer in 1895, it focuses on the mechanical 'fixations' in the spine. Because this is the home of the central nervous system, these can cause problems throughout the body.

Methods of treatment 'Fixations' have many causes – injury, disease, allergy, stress or poor posture – and are treated by 'mobilisation' – moving the joint surfaces apart. This is done with the person lying on a couch, and most people say it is not painful.

Length of treatment Dealing with the initial problem may take only a handful of relatively short sessions but most chiropractors recommend regular visits.

Attitudes of medical doctors Generally positive, as the benefits of chiropractic can be demonstrated through research.

Regulatory body The British Chiropractic Association (address on p 150). A statutory body regulating chiropractic, the General Chiropractic Council (address on p 154), was established in 1999.

Western herbal medicine

Western herbal medicine – the forerunner of mainstream medicine – is recommended by its practitioners for most conditions, including arthritis, and particularly for stress, gastro-intestinal, menstrual and hormonal problems.

Basic principles The therapeutic use of herbs is as old as human beings. The Western tradition, which is based on Greek and Roman principles, sees the herbs as stimulating the body's healing process although many of their properties – anti-bacterial, anti-viral and so on – are much as mainstream synthetic drugs. Indeed, although herbal medicines are 'natural', they can be even more toxic than drugs so it is not a good idea to self-prescribe anything stronger than a herbal tea.

Methods of treatment Very full case histories are taken and often a physical examination is involved before a personalised herbal formula is prescribed.

Length of treatment One visit may be sufficient, although this is less likely with a complex condition such as arthritis.

Attitudes of medical doctors Not generally dismissive, as herbs are the basis of many modern drugs (eg aspirin contains a substance found in willow bark), but tend to be concerned about the difficulties of getting a precise dose from a natural and therefore variable product. This is worth discussing with your herbalist.

Regulatory body The National Institute of Medical Herbalists (address on p 157). Look out for the initials MNIMH.

Chinese herbal medicine

Chinese herbal medicine is recommended by its practitioners for most conditions, including arthritis, for which, in China, it remains the most popular treatment even though Western medicine is now available there too.

Basic principles Chinese medicine, based on the principle of balance mentioned under acupuncture, is some 23 centuries old. It sees herbs – which are categorised according to their nature (eg hot or cold), taste and the particular organ they enter – as restoring the imbalances that cause disease.

Methods of treatment Pills or extracts are the most likely treatment for a chronic condition such as arthritis, and dietary suggestions may well be made. The approach is holistic, treating the whole person not just the problem presented.

Length of treatment More than one visit is likely to be needed, and, in general, treatments are slower acting than Western drugs.

Attitude of medical doctors Tend to be unenthusiastic despite the fact that some Chinese remedies have proved effective in trials. As with Western herbal medicine, there are concerns over getting a precise dose and occasional reports of serious ill-effects.

Regulatory body None, but many Chinese-trained practitioners are members of the Association of Traditional Chinese Medicine (address on p 149). Look out also for the Register of Chinese Herbal Medicine (RCHM).

Homoeopathy

Homoeopathy is recommended by its practitioners for most conditions, although homoeopaths would suggest an osteopath or chiropractor for structural problems.

Basic principles Founded by the German doctor Samuel Hahnemann in the eighteenth century, it is based on the principle that like cures like. An immeasurably small amount of the substance that causes the problem is used to stimulate the body's own healing mechanisms.

Methods of treatment A detailed personal history will be taken. Medicines – usually a single remedy – are generally given in small sugary tablets.

Length of treatment Sessions may be long, especially the first one. With a chronic condition such as arthritis, several sessions over some time may be required.

Attitudes of medical doctors Homoeopathy is available on the NHS, and there is research to suggest that it does work in some cases. However, nobody can explain satisfactorily why it works, given that the dilutions in the dose are so great that, according to the laws of physics, the original is no longer measurably present.

Regulatory body There are two, the Society of Homoeopaths and the British Homoeopathic Association (addresses on p 159 and p 150). Members of the latter organisation are also trained doctors.

Massage

Massage is recommended by its practitioners for anybody at all, and specifically for aches and pains related to stress and muscle tension.

Basic principles We all know the benefit of touch. That's why we rub the spot when we hurt ourselves. Massage helps eliminate toxins, stimulate the flow of blood and lymph, and soothe the nerves. There are two types: remedial and relaxation.

Methods of treatment The client will be asked what sort of massage is required – vigorous and stimulating or gentle and relaxing – and if any parts of the body are to be avoided (eg an inflamed joint). Clothes are removed and towels used to cover the body. These are removed and replaced as each part of the body is worked on – the masseur rubbing, kneading and stimulating the body as required. Massage is often combined with aromatherapy, and all masseurs will use oils or talcum powder. A massage must be stopped if it is painful.

Length of treatment As required; massage is a feel-good treatment rather than a remedy.

Attitudes of medical doctors Positive, so long as it's done carefully. Some hospitals now make massage available to patients.

Regulatory body None, although lists of qualified masseurs and aromatherapy masseurs are available from the Institute for Complementary Medicine (address on p 155).

Osteopathy

Osteopathy is recommended by its practitioners for anything structural, including arthritis.

Basic principles Founded in 1874 by American doctor Andrew Taylor Still, a Christian who believed that if we are created in God's image then all faults in our functioning must arise from the way we use our bodies. Osteopaths attempt to right these misalignments to allow the bodily fluids and nerves to work correctly.

Methods of treatment The person lies on a couch while the osteopath makes 'adjustments' and relaxes the soft tissues to allow the body to heal itself. Most people find it relaxing and not painful.

Length of treatment This will depend on the problem. With arthritis, regular visits may be suggested. The osteopath will usually say how many treatments will be needed to achieve a result.

Attitudes of medical doctors Generally positive, as they are for chiropractic.

Regulatory body The General Osteopathic Council (address on p 155).

Reflexology

Reflexology is recommended by its practitioners for anybody, but particularly for aches and pains, immune system problems, stress and lack of energy.

Basic principles There are indications that there was something like reflexology in ancient Eastern cultures but its modern father is American ear, nose and throat specialist William H Fitzgerald. He discovered that pressure applied to one part of the body could relieve pain in another. Using this principle, a reflexologist accesses the whole body – which is divided into zones – from the foot. Massage here can unblock energy flows between zones and promote healing.

Methods of treatment Pressure with the practitioner's thumb to the person's foot and sometimes hand. It's too firm to tickle but may be slightly painful as 'blockages' are released. Most people feel good after a treatment.

Length of treatment Perhaps once every six weeks or so.

Attitudes of medical doctors Most acknowledge the benefit of a foot massage though few accept reflexology's full analysis. Physiotherapists and occupational therapists are usually more enthusiastic.

Regulatory body None, but the largest independent organisation is the Association of Reflexologists (address on p 149). The initials MAR indicate that the therapist has a qualification in reflexology.

Yoga

Yoga is recommended by its practitioners for anybody to improve posture, muscle tone and flexibility and to help relaxation.

Basic principles Ancient Eastern, particularly Indian. The various positions (or asanas) adopted in yoga have evolved over thousands of years. By moving the body in different ways and directions they stimulate muscles and joints and help the circulation and the flow of bodily fluids.

Methods of treatment Yoga is not strictly a therapy, because nobody practices on anyone. Many books are available, but the best way to learn the asanas and the breathing and meditation techniques that can accompany them is from a teacher. Classes are run at most adult education and leisure centres. People with arthritis should avoid straining to reach a position and must make sure that the teacher knows of their condition, as some positions may be inappropriate. A therapeutic yoga teacher may be able to provide a customised programme.

Attitudes of medical doctors Be careful with your joints.

Regulatory body There are many types of yoga and no single regulatory body. My yoga teacher suggests the Iyengar Institute or the gentler British Wheel of Yoga.

Other therapies

Where no governing body is listed or for information on other therapies, contact the Institute for Complementary Medicine (address on p 155).

For more *i*nformation

i For more information about complementary therapy, contact the listed regulatory body or the Institute for Complementary Medicine (addresses in the 'Useful addresses' section at the back of this book).

i The issues considered here will be covered in much more detail in any good self-help book. Two worth considering include my book *Getting a Grip – Self-help for arthritis and rheumatism* (out of print now but may be available at your local library) and *The Arthritis Helpbook* by Kate Lorig and James Fries. These also consider some of the issues not covered here such as developing your social life and personal relationships when you have arthritis.

3 What should you do?

This chapter discusses frankly the challenges that caring brings, and aims to help you decide what best to do. It looks at what it is like to be cared for, whether you should consider becoming a carer and what rights you will have if you do.

Sheena

'Last year we were given a shop for the day for Carers National Association at our local shopping mall. We made lots of posters – all by hand – and put them in the shop. We went there first thing in the morning, started putting balloons up and getting ready, and when we looked there was a queue right the way down the shopping mall of people waiting to come in.

'They couldn't wait for us to open, to ask all these questions. It was incredible. You can't believe the people who are out there. It was carers listening to other carers. Some carers are frightened to go and talk to anybody official. They feel that they might lose their pensions or their little bit of money, or the help that they've got. But they were only too happy to come in and discuss it with us. Because really – let's face it – we, other carers, are the true professionals.'

Are you a carer already? The Carers National Association define a carer as follows:

'You're a carer if your life is in any way restricted by the need to provide care at home for someone who can't manage without your help. And the reason they can't manage might be old age, disability, some kind of mental or physical ill health. But the key thing is you are absolutely necessary to their ability to cope at home. That might mean that you're doing it for a short time, a few hours a week only. Or it might mean, and it does mean this for many carers, that you're caring seven days a week, twenty-four hours a day, for ten, fifteen, twenty years.'

It's easy to slide along the scale – a few hours become a few more hours become a few days. This may well be the right way for you to go but it is important to do it with your eyes open. When you are considering what you should do for your relative or friend or partner with arthritis, the first thing to think about is: what is it like to be cared for?

What is it like to be cared for?

There is no doubt that being a carer can be hard work. But being cared for also has its problems and frustrations.

Maria

'It's not easy being "cared for". It's not just the messy bits. It's no longer being able to nick a chocolate biscuit out of the fridge, or experiment with make-up, or grab just the right scarf to set off your jumper as you rush out the door. Always, always, you have to ask.

'These things may seem insignificant nit-pickings compared with the more obviously dramatic changes wrought by disability, but taken together they are momentous. As they are given up, a little bit of what outwardly makes you an individual is eroded.

'No one would deny that looking after another person can be tough. It is also often a job reluctantly undertaken. Knowing all this, reading all the accounts of ruined lives, it can be just as tough finding yourself in the position of having to receive all this "care" – your self-esteem can easily be drowned out by guilt and gratefulness. If carers are way down the ladder then those they care for are at the bottom, popularly seen as tyrants, as indifferent to their helper's feelings as pampered pet poodles.'

What is caring?

'Caring' is a nice word – we all like to think we care – but it's tough work emotionally, physically and financially. Just what are you taking on if you become someone's carer?

It is important to distinguish between caring *about* and caring *for*. Caring about each other has got to be a good thing – the world needs more of it. Caring for someone is more complicated. It's what we do for those who can't do it for themselves. To be cared for is something that all adults need and enjoy from time to time but few would want *all* of the time. I don't. I doubt that you do. And most people with arthritis don't – certainly not in my experience of working with them. So you need to bear this fact in mind: if you choose to become another adult's carer you are becoming something they would rather not have. For this reason it should be a fall-back position – a plan B (or even plan C, D or E) – rather than a first choice. If you care about someone (in the first sense of the word), you'll want to give them what we all want: as much independence as possible for as long as possible.

Be clear what being a carer involves. Many carers provide personal help with toileting and bathing, for example, and with physically demanding tasks such as lifting and washing. In the case of arthritis, there can also be a lot of small but frequent tasks such as opening bottle tops or turning taps on or off. Seven in ten carers in a Carers National Association survey put in more than 100 hours of caring a week. As many as two-thirds had health problems of their own.

Despite the Carers (Recognition and Services) Act 1995, which was intended to enshrine carers' rights, their situation may actually be deteriorating. The Crossroads Care organisation, which represents some 230 carer support schemes, reckon they are supporting more carers who are caring on less income. The Carers National Association estimate that the 7 million carers in the UK save the nation around £34 billion a year but it is work that is seldom recognised by the rest of us and certainly not adequately by the state. Listen to Hilary, who cares for a friend with fibrositis.

Hilary

'I would like to see carers who are looking after a relative or friend accorded the same financial and professional treatment as the social services provide care assistants. If you're a carer on Income Support you can, in some cases, get a premium but it's just £15 a week compared to £4 an hour for a care assistant. Getting grants is harder, too. Most applications need a social worker's recommendation but if you're a private carer you might not have a social worker. This is my second time as a carer and it's harder the second time around because you know more about what you may have to do and you know how little help you're going to get to do it. If official bodies know what a carer is, you're lucky – although this is improving now.'

The concern with money isn't penny-pinching. It's reality for many carers. Fifty per cent of carers give up work to provide care, say the Carers National Association. And it can be a full-time job.

Hilary again

'It's not easy to switch off. You don't have your own life unless the person you're caring for is out of the house or with someone you trust. Otherwise, every second, you're aware of what they're doing. If the person you care for can't go out much, neither can you.

'I'm fortunate to be on the Internet so I can 'go out' from inside my own home. I monitor a carers' news group but I also use it to talk about other things. It stops me feeling alienated from the world. I think it's that alienation that non-carers find hard to understand. The thing is that, when you love the person you're caring for, you can't just walk away. How do you turn round and say "I'm sorry, I can't cope with you"?'

In short, caring involves giving a lot. Some people are better suited temperamentally to this than others; some are even attracted to it, and the system certainly relies on this. However, if you give up your own life for another, you are not necessarily doing them a favour. If your own health breaks down, you will no longer be able to provide them with the same service while at the same time their guilt and resentment will grow – guilt over what you're doing for them and the damage it is doing to you and resentment over the degree of control you have over their lives. You may feel guilt and resentment too – guilt over what you are not doing for them and resentment over what you do.

If you doubt that this will happen to you, think seriously about why you are considering becoming a carer. Is it because you feel sorry for the other person? Is it a sense of duty? Is it out of love? All three probably, if you're honest with yourself. Duty and sympathy, even if tempered with the strongest of love, can conjure up guilt and resentment sooner or later. You should not feel bad about the negative feelings you will at times have towards the person for whom you care. Sometimes they'll be very strong. And don't kid yourself that you won't have them, because you will not find a carer who hasn't had them at some point. Better to have thought about it and, ideally, have talked about it in advance. Better still to have explored options for independence and professional caring first.

Control is a key issue. Caring should be a supportive role, not a decision-making one. For this reason, many disabled people prefer the term 'personal assistant' to 'carer', because this term makes it far clearer where the decisions are made. You are there to help the person you are caring for to live the life they want to, not to decide what sort of life that should be. This can be very difficult because they will, at some point, make a decision that you don't like or agree with. That much is guaranteed.

If you do become a carer, it is important that you have an outlet for the negative feelings you will experience. You don't want to take them out on the person you are caring for but you must not bottle them up.

Caroline

'I was caring for my husband, Jeff (who had arthritis), working full-time as a teacher and bringing up a son. I had no relatives and felt it was all on my shoulders. I felt very responsible. The inevitable happened. My job became so stressful that I took early retirement, my asthma was terrible and I was diagnosed with depression. I saw a counsellor and it was she who pointed out just what I was taking on. The thing is I was feeling guilty about my negative feelings, which was no good. You have to let them out or you'll get depressed. You're not a horrible person for having horrible feelings. If you feel angry, it's because you've got a lot to be angry about. Look after yourself.

'Before Jeff died, I apologised for all the harsh things I'd said to him and he said he understood. As a carer, you don't just need information, you need support – from other carers and, I think, from a professional counsellor – a safe confidential place where you can say all those things you're ashamed about feeling.'

So, before getting into the ins and outs of everyday caring, it's important to have a clear idea of your role as a carer. The needs of the person you are caring for must be your focus. That means the needs they express, not the needs you believe they have. Of course, if the person's health prevents them from expressing their needs then that is a different situation but this is not the case with a physical disability such as arthritis.

This means that your relationship with the person should be such that they feel comfortable about expressing their true feelings with you, and you with them. Few relationships enjoy that degree of frankness – we often, for the best of motives, protect the ones we love from our real feelings. It's far easier to be blunt with a professional carer. A relationship will change when one party begins to care for (rather than care about) the other. It has to. It will challenge even the most loving relationship.

Jenny

'I was still at school when Mum first got bad, and the role reversal was very stressful. It affected my exams. Helping with personal tasks is tough for us both. I feel that her loss of dignity is in some ways worse for her because I'm her daughter.

'My advice is to get help as soon as possible. Mum has an occupational therapist now who helps a lot with equipment and a home help three times a week, but she's really had to fight for everything.'

If you become a carer, it must be your choice. There are alternatives, as this book will show. 'I *had* to' is not a good enough reason – you owe it to yourself and the person you are caring for to have thought about it more thoroughly than that.

My mum says that my grandfather used to say to her 'You only have children so they can look after you in your old age', and he was only partly joking. It was clear what he expected and, in due course, she did look after him. She has made it equally clear that she doesn't expect the same from me or my brother – not least because of the difficulties it caused her. So ideas of family obligation vary with our own upbringing and attitude – they are not fixed. You do *not* have to do it.

Think creatively. Maximise the options that maintain the other person's independence, rather than helping them too much. In truth, the best carer may not be someone with the traditional caring skills but someone who is assertive and knows their rights and those of the person they are caring for. The health service and local and central government do have caring roles and responsibilities – the best service you can give may be to ensure that these roles and responsibilities are taken.

Carers' rights

However clearly you see your role as a carer (and it is important that you *do* see it clearly), your role in the eyes of the state and society in general will probably be unclear. Some people still see caring as the natural extension of a family relationship, and for a long time governments have thought the same.

When he was piloting through Parliament the Private Member's Bill that became the Carers (Recognition and Services) Act, Malcolm Wicks was blunt about how carers are seen by themselves and others. He said that carers are:

'taken for granted by the welfare state, taken for granted by social workers and doctors, and not given the support that they need. Often the GP or the social worker visiting is almost literally patting the person on the back, saying: "You're doing a great job, keep going". Instead of saying: "Hang on a minute, how are you? When did you last have a good night's sleep? When did you have a break? Is there anything we can do for you?" And that's the mentality that we've got to change round.'

This has changed a little, and the Carers (Recognition and Services) Act – often called just the Carers Act – which came into force in 1996, clarifies what carers can expect. Promoted by the Carers National Association, it says that:

- Carers have a right to ask for a social services assessment of their ability to care – previously only the person being cared for could be assessed.
- Local authorities have a duty to take into account the results of this assessment when looking at what support to provide for the person being cared for.

The Act covers three groups of carers:

- adults who care for other adults;
- those who care for ill or disabled children under 19;
- young people under 18 who care for a relative.

Only carers who are providing 'regular and substantial' care are eligible for assessments, and only if the person for whom they care is receiving an assessment or re-assessment. (Social services assessments are covered in detail on pages 88–90.)

The problem is that sometimes social services workers are reluctant to do an assessment when they feel that the resources available will be unable to deliver the services that might be needed. They might not volunteer the information that you are entitled to an assessment too, even if they do assess the person for whom you care. Make sure you ask for one. Don't wait until you hit a crisis to ask for help. Ask social services what carers' assessment practice they are following, and if you can have a copy of the policy and an assessment form. Ask who is in charge of carers' assessments. The Carers National Association have produced good practice guidelines for assessing carers. Ask your social services department if they follow them.

Of course, you won't go in all guns blazing – social and health services staff *do* want to help – but be prepared for what might be a long, hard struggle in some cases. You may have to keep asking, and perhaps even fight for it, but there is help available, as the next chapter will show.

For further *i*nformation

i *Choices for the carer of an elderly relative* by Marina Lewycka, published by Age Concern Books.

i *The Carer's Handbook: What to do and who to turn to* by Marina Lewycka, published by Age Concern Books.

i Age Concern Factsheet 6 *Finding help at home.*

i Perhaps the best source of further information on this is other carers, particularly those among your friends and family whom you can talk to honestly about your concerns and those in your area who can advise you of what is available locally. Contact Carers National Association (address on p 150).

4 Who can help?

The most important person in the management of arthritis is the person who has it. Nevertheless, there are a whole range of other people it is sensible to involve, the most obvious being the health professionals.

This chapter outlines where you can go for help – health and social services professionals, voluntary organisations and the family. Also discussed are suggestions for getting the best out of them. Making sure that service providers are aware of your needs and those of the person you are caring for is a key part of the challenge.

Caroline

'The GP is your gateway to local authority and other support. Try to find a GP who understands your role. Be honest with your GP. State what you need, don't wait for it to be offered, and keep asking.'

General practitioner (GP)

Everybody has the right to be registered with a GP – the first port of call for any illness, including a carer's.

Finding a GP

It has been estimated by Arthritis Care and the Arthritis Research Campaign that at least one in five GP appointments concerns arthritis, so a good relationship between a person with arthritis and their GP is very important. Similarly, make sure your own GP knows all about your caring responsibilities, so it will be easier for them to notice if these affect your health. It is possible that you too have some arthritis yourself, so take this opportunity to learn about managing it effectively. Don't wait until the condition becomes a serious problem.

When you register with a new GP, you should, under the Patient's Charter, be offered an introductory health check. This may well be repeated annually for patients who are 75 or over. If it is not offered, ask. Also ask for information about the services the practice offers and whether it has its own practice charter. The charter will outline what you can expect from the practice: opening times, facilities for disabled people and children, arrangements for tests and repeat prescriptions, and so on.

People with arthritis tend to need the assistance of a broad range of health professionals, so the more services a GP practice can provide – physiotherapy, counselling, practice nurse and so on – the better. A 'one-stop shop' makes referral easier and reduces travelling. Familiarity enables better relationships to be built. For this reason a larger multi-doctor practice or health centre is probably your best bet.

You may be unable to register with the local GP of your choice – they may already have too many patients, for example – or you may want to change your GP (the Patient's Charter says that you have the right to change 'easily and quickly if you want to'). If so, contact your local health authority, who will provide you with a full list of general practices in your area.

It could be worth trying to find one of the 400 GPs who are members of the Primary Care Rheumatology Society, an organisation for family doctors with a special interest in arthritis. Ask your GP whether they are a member. If they are not, encourage them to join.

Remember that most carers have, or develop, their own health problems. Don't ignore them. You need to take care of yourself if you are to take care of someone else. See your own GP sooner rather than later if you have any problems.

What can the GP offer?

Many people with arthritis feel there is little that a GP can do for them. This is not so. GPs monitor drugs, suggest other forms of treatment and advise on exercise, diet and anything else the patient might like to try.

In most cases of arthritis, the GP will be up against a disease that is difficult to diagnose, affects different people in different ways and for which there are treatments but no cures. A tough challenge. Time is an important factor in the diagnosis of arthritis but the symptoms such as pain, swelling and fatigue need immediate treatment. So, a prescription without a full explanation may well be the initial response. That's all right at first but don't put up with it for too long.

Referral

A very important thing that a GP can do is provide a referral to specialists. Joint pain is the biggest single reason for referral to hospital, so a request should not be refused.

The Patient's Charter says that a patient has the right to 'be referred to a consultant acceptable to you, when your GP thinks it is necessary, and to be referred for a second opinion if you and your GP agree this is desirable'. After referral, nine out of ten patients should be seen within 13 weeks, according to the Charter. Since the abolition of the internal market in the NHS, GPs should no longer have to worry about having sufficient funds for referral.

In April 1999, primary care groups (GPs, dentists, etc) took financial responsibility for planning and funding health services for the communities they serve. Primary care groups are charged with improving the health of the local population, improving local primary and community services, and commissioning hospital services for local patients. Primary care groups are run by a board consisting of GPs, nurses, a social services officer, a health authority representative and a local member of the public.

Nobody is obliged to see a consultant – many people with arthritis manage their disease with their GP alone – but it makes sense to take advantage of a specialist's greater knowledge and hospital facilities. Anybody whose arthritis is sufficiently severe that they have care needs that can only be met by someone else should see a consultant. Everyone with suspected rheumatoid arthritis, ankylosing spondylitis or vasculitis should press to see a consultant, even if this means travelling some distance.

Hospital consultant

Hospital consultants who specialise in arthritis and rheumatic diseases are called rheumatologists. Although they will use many of the diagnostic techniques discussed in Chapter 2, they will know more about the disease than a GP and be more familiar with its many variations. The consultant rheumatologist is usually the leader of a team that will take overall responsibility for treatment. They may also refer on to another health or community professional or, in some cases, to an orthopaedic surgeon who specialises in joint replacement and other surgery.

The Royal College of Physicians estimates that there should be one rheumatologist for every 150,000 people. The NHS falls some way short of this. A study in 1993 by the charity Arthritis Research Campaign (then the Arthritis and Rheumatism Council for Research) found that Portugal and Eire were the only European countries with a lower ratio of rheumatologists per head of population than the UK. The differences are striking. For example, Denmark had 3.4 rheumatologists per 100,000 people whereas the UK had 0.6. In the UK, Northern Ireland, Scotland and Wales tend to be less well served than England. For this reason it can take a long wait and possibly a long journey to see a rheumatologist.

Surgery

Operations for arthritis include joint replacement, joint fusion, removal of inflamed tissue, removal of some bone to ease pain, repair of damage to tendons, and release of a trapped nerve.

Replacements are usually offered if the joint has become very badly damaged and is not responding to other treatment. The most common is a hip replacement, although knees, ankles, shoulders, elbows and joints in the wrists and fingers can also be replaced. The joint is removed under anaesthetic and replaced with an artificial one, called a prosthesis, made from plastic and metal. Since June 1998, all prostheses have had to meet a European standard, although testing is still not as rigorous as for a new drug.

According to Arthritis Care, over 40,000 hips are replaced every year in the UK. The Arthritis Research Campaign anticipate that this figure will rise to over 50,000 in the next few years. The vast majority of hip replacements leave the patient without pain and with three-quarters of 'normal' mobility in the joint. A modern prosthesis can last 15 years or more but should be checked regularly using X-ray and physical examination. Some 10–20 per cent of hip replacements are 'revisions' (ie repeat operations). Knees are the second most commonly replaced joint.

Replacements used to be 'saved' for patients over 60 but now younger people are also likely to be offered one. Surgery is not inevitable in arthritis but it can revolutionise one's quality of life. Someone whose arthritis is sufficiently severe that they have care needs that can only be met by somebody else is the sort of patient who is more likely to be offered surgery or, indeed, to ask for it. It's always the patient's choice to proceed.

The key questions when considering surgery are:

- What exactly is being offered?
- What are the benefits?
- What should be possible afterwards that is not possible now?
- What will not be possible?
- What are the risks? (These are small but include infection,

thrombosis, dislocation of the joint and, in a very tiny number of cases, death.)

■ Who will do the surgery and what experience do they have?

■ What prosthesis will be used and what is its track record like?

Surgeons are not robots. Some are better than others. A surgeon who performs a specific operation once or twice a year is unlikely to be as experienced, and therefore as competent, as a surgeon who performs the same procedure 30 times. Common sense suggests that the more common a type of surgery, the greater the likelihood that the surgeon performing it is experienced, but it makes sense to talk to your surgeon about their record and expertise as well as with other patients, friendly doctors, the theatre sister or the relevant business manager in the hospital. At present, surgeons' records are not published but organisations such as the College of Health are campaigning for it.

It is extremely valuable to talk to someone else who has had the operation. Such people may be found through the hospital but the best bet is probably a local group of Arthritis Care or a local disability organisation. The Arthritis Care helpline can provide an information sheet as well as useful advice about how best to prepare for and recover from the operation. Hospitals often provide this too, but the standard of their written information sometimes falls far below that recommended by the British League Against Rheumatism.

Kate Llewellyn was 25 when she had her knee replaced. She told *Arthritis News*:

Kate

'It has been ten months since my operation and I can't stop raving about my knee. It is amazing – free of pain and it bends to over 95 degrees.'

But it's not plain sailing.

Kate again

'The first week post-op was not pleasant. The pain-killing regimen made me very ill and didn't work. My saviours were the physiotherapists, despite the weeks of pain they put me through. It was they who made my new knee work.'

Author Leslie Thomas has had both hips replaced. He says quite simply that they've changed his life.

Leslie

'It knocked the stuffing out of me for six months but it was the best thing I've ever done and I'd have no hesitation about doing it again. The only thing is, I still can't get out of the bath. I play cricket again now, a couple of sets of tennis, although I can't walk far enough to play golf.'

The Department of Health says nobody should wait longer than 18 months for a hip or knee replacement. The College of Health runs the National Waiting List Helpline (020 8983 1133) which can sometimes help patients find a shorter waiting list than the one they have been referred to.

Hip replacements can be carried out privately. If you are tempted by this option, don't be swayed by niceties such as a private room or an exotic menu; check out the things that really matter. Ask about the experience and expertise of the surgeon very carefully. If you will be in a private hospital, ask about the quality and amount of nursing care, and what will happen if anything goes wrong. Don't assume that private health care will get you better treatment than on the NHS.

Physiotherapist (physio)

A patient can be referred for physiotherapy by their GP or consultant, or can pay for it privately. Some larger GP practices may have a visiting physiotherapist. Otherwise, it may be necessary to attend the hospital physiotherapy department. For physiotherapy, it is unlikely that referral will be to any hospital other than the local one but it doesn't hurt to ask.

Hospital physiotherapists are usually generalists rather than specialists. For the more common forms of arthritis with 'typical' mobility problems they should be fine. Otherwise, it can sometimes be a bit of a lottery. Quality and expertise vary within departments, so it can be worth asking to see someone with experience of the specific type of arthritis.

Having the 'right' physiotherapist is important because their work is often crucial in the treatment of arthritis. They concentrate on relieving pain and improving mobility of the joints using manipulation and treatments such as ultrasound (which stimulates the body tissue using inaudible, high-frequency sound waves), ice-packs and heat. They will probably suggest exercises to be done at home, most of which might seem so simple that it can be difficult to believe that they will work. In fact, they are highly effective and well worth the effort.

A typical course of treatment will last about ten sessions. Most hospitals are reluctant to offer longer term care because of the cost. For a long-term condition such as arthritis, this is not helpful.

Private physiotherapy is worth considering for more specialised or intensive help. For names of local private physiotherapists, contact the Chartered Society of Physiotherapy. See only a physiotherapist who is a member of the Society and who understands both arthritis in general and the needs of the person you are caring for in particular.

In some areas, hydrotherapy may be available. This is physiotherapy in the water, done under the supervision of physiotherapists.

Most people find that it helps their arthritis and virtually everyone enjoys it. The hydrotherapy pool is lovely and warm, and special equipment (eg lifting devices) is available so that even the most severely disabled people can benefit.

Joy

'I used to do hydrotherapy every week for about 20 minutes. A senior physiotherapist helped with the exercises. It's amazing how much exercise you can do in the lovely warm water that you can't do on land. The problem is that it's not available everywhere on the NHS; even where it is, it's usually only for a short time. Our Arthritis Care group hired the hydro pool so we could all go regularly – we took 30 to 40 people.'

From Getting a Grip: Self-help for arthritis *by Jim Pollard; Headline 1996*

Occupational therapist (OT)

The occupational therapist is a health professional a carer really needs to know about, because they can make a real difference and may become a long-term ally for you and the person you are caring for. An occupational therapist will discuss with the person with arthritis their day-to-day activities, and can then advise about any aids or gadgets that might be helpful or even suggest structural alterations to the home. It is very important to tell the occupational therapist about what can*not* be done – it is surprising how many difficulties can be overcome with a little imagination. Sometimes the occupational therapist may be limited to merely making recommendations, so you may have to do some lobbying as well to get them implemented.

The objective is to enable the person with arthritis to do as many everyday tasks as possible, as easily as possible while protecting their joints as much as possible. Simply rearranging the home or adjusting the way something is gripped or lifted may make a significant difference – and at no cost.

Occupational therapists work either as part of the hospital rheumatology team or for the social services. Those based in the hospital usually do splinting and arrange for the loan of equipment to be used at home; those from social services are generally concerned with a person's coping abilities and can recommend household equipment such as rising chairs, ramps and stairlifts. Social services occupational therapists are usually contacted by referral from the doctor; sometimes, though, from reluctance, ignorance or absent-mindedness, doctors may not refer as often as they could. Insist. Alternatively, contact one through your social services department. (There is more about social services on p 87.)

Pharmacist

Pharmacists can give advice about the medicines that the person you care for needs, whether they are on prescription or bought over the counter. Some pharmacist/chemist shops have a prescription collection and delivery service or they may make home visits. Many have a computer database that can print out information about any specific drug.

Helping someone get the best out of a health professional

■ Ask the person you are caring for if they would like you to accompany them to an appointment, and respect their right to say 'no'.
■ If you do go together, offer practical support such as taking notes or running a cassette recorder.

■ Discuss beforehand what they hope to get out of the appointment and what specific questions they want answered. Gently remind them of these during the consultation if necessary.

■ Discuss with them how they will answer the more obvious questions but do not, during the consultation, answer for them. Resist any attempts the professional might make to talk to you rather than the patient.

■ Try to encourage the person you are caring for to say more if you feel they are trivialising their arthritis or worrying about wasting the professional's time. Encourage the professional to say more if they are not speaking plainly.

■ Talk to health professionals as you would a genuine friend, even if they don't feel like one.

■ Arthritis Care produces good practice guidelines for primary health care (GPs, etc) and secondary health care (hospitals). Make sure the health professionals you deal with have copies.

Kate Lorig, Director of Patient Education Research at Stanford Arthritis Center in the USA, believes that the good patient should be a CAD: 'Come prepared. Ask questions. Discuss problems.' This technique can be applied equally well to your appointments with all health professionals or complementary therapists.

Social services and community care

A person with arthritis may be entitled to assistance under community care legislation. Help may be available at home with the following:

■ home care (eg cooking, shopping or more personal tasks such as dressing);

■ meals-on-wheels;

■ aids and equipment (eg a hand-rail for the bath);

■ counselling;

■ occupational therapy;

■ night sitting;

■ help with holidays;

- help with transport;
- help with installing a telephone.

Respite care and temporary residential or nursing home care may also be available, to give you a break from caring.

Local authorities have an obligation to help in these ways under a number of Acts of Parliament, including the Health Services and Public Health Act 1968, the Chronically Sick and Disabled Persons Act 1970, the National Health Service Act 1977 and the Mental Health Act 1983 as well as the National Health Service and Community Care Act 1990. In practice, the degree of help given is limited by the resources available. However, the statutory obligation remains, creating what can be a complex legal situation. If you feel harshly or unfairly treated, don't give up. Read this section carefully and then reapply, appeal or take further advice.

Community care is arranged through the local authority's social services department. In most parts of England and Wales, social services comes under the county council or unitary authority; in London it is the metropolitan or borough council. In Scotland it is under the regional council, and in Northern Ireland under the local health and social services board or trust.

Getting the best out of a community care assessment

The first step is to make an appointment with the social services or social work department for an assessment to determine 'needs'. They have an obligation to assess:

- anyone who is disabled;
- anyone who helps to look after someone else – in which case both persons' needs should be assessed;
- anyone else who seems to have needs.

The local authority must assess anyone with any need for a service which it has the power to provide (ie those listed on p 87), even if it does not provide that service at the time. If a person is disabled, the local authority must offer an assessment for services specified in section 2 of the Chronically Sick and Disabled Persons Act 1970 and the Disabled Persons (Services, Representation and Consultation)

Act 1986. A reassessment should be requested whenever a person's needs change.

Under the legislation, a person is deemed to be disabled if they are 'blind, deaf or dumb (or who suffer from mental disorder of any description) and other persons aged 18 or over who are substantially or permanently handicapped by illness, injury or congenital deformity or such other disabilities as may be prescribed by the Secretary of State' (National Assistance Act 1948, section 29) or, under more recent government guidance, someone who is partially sighted or hard of hearing. A disabled person, so defined, has greater rights to services than someone who does not fit the definition. Registration of disability for the purpose of employment is not an issue. Anybody whose arthritis is so severe that they have care needs should be covered by this definition.

The local authority should publish a community care charter explaining its procedures, including such information as how long one should have to wait for an assessment. The assessment – which is free – should be carried out by a social worker, occupational therapist, social services care manager, health visitor or other professional but there is no national standard. The assessment interview can take place in the person's home, in hospital or in a council office. The person being assessed can have a friend or relative with them; this is a good idea for moral support and to act as an aide memoire.

Caroline, a carer who has lots of experience in both carers' and disabled people's organisations, says it is important to be absolutely frank.

Caroline

'Make sure they know what you *can't* do – not what you can. The definition of something you can't do is simple. If you cannot do it every day as often as you want without help, however small that help might be, then you cannot do it. Don't put on a brave face. In my experience you cannot be brave *and* get what you want.'

Needs could be written down and a copy given to the interviewer. Consider every aspect of living – getting up, washing, going to the toilet and bathing, dressing, cleaning, getting around the house, cooking, laundry, shopping, paying bills and completing forms, going out, taking holidays, companionship and so on. Make sure that every difficulty is included, however trivial it may seem.

Local authorities are making a determined effort to develop 'user-centred' services that respond flexibly to the specific needs of people and give them increased choice. So be clear about needs. Assessors may attempt to put people in boxes that match the services they know are available. Don't accept this. The 1998 White Paper *Modernising Social Services* says that services should be adapted to provide what people need, not the other way round.

Most local authorities charge for the community care services they provide, but this charge should be reasonable and should not be more than it costs the council to provide them. If the person cannot afford to pay in full, the local authority should undertake a financial assessment to find out what it is reasonable for that individual to pay. This financial assessment should always take place *after* the assessment of needs.

After the assessment, the interviewer should list the individual's needs in writing and give them a copy. Social services will then specify which services they can offer to meet those needs and at what cost. This will be called a 'care package' or a 'care plan'. There is a right of appeal – both about the type of care being offered and about the cost – and in most cases the individual can turn down any services they do not want.

Penny

'I found that I lived in a fairly open-minded authority – they included independent living in their provision. At that time social services could provide 40 hours a week of help from personal (care) assistants. And I got a car through Motability.'

The assessment should also identify unmet needs – needs that exist but which the local authority cannot meet.

The individual may not get or be entitled to all the services they want. In this case, ask what the local authority's assessment criteria are. All local authorities have thresholds or other criteria that they use to decide who should receive a certain service and who should not, although some may deny this. Criteria often change in April – the beginning of a new financial year. If the individual does not get what they need, there are three options: appeal, legal action or find other sources of help. In all cases it is worth seeking assistance from a law centre, advice bureau, community health council or the disability organisation RADAR. Remember to keep copies of all letters you send and make a note of every phone call, including the name of the person you spoke to.

Appeal The local authority's community care charter should include an explanation of its appeals process (often also called the complaints process). Cases of maladministration (such as neglect, unjustifiable delay, unfair discrimination or failure to have the proper procedures or to abide by them) can be taken to the Local Government Ombudsman and/or to the Local Government Monitoring Officer (a senior local authority official). The local authority will provide names and addresses for both of these. Ultimately, an appeal can be made to the Secretary of State.

Legal action If the local authority's action is unlawful, it may be possible, as a last resort, to sue them for breach of statutory duty but this is hard to prove. It is worth bringing any action of the local authority that might be unlawful to the attention of the Monitoring Officer, who is there to see that the authority acts within the law. An alternative is to ask the High Court for a judicial review if the local authority has behaved illegally, irrationally or failed to follow the correct procedures. If you are considering this, talk first to someone at a law centre, advice bureau or specialist disability organisation, and certainly to your MP.

Find alternative sources of help This is discussed on pages 94–98.

Direct payments

For many disabled people, direct payment is the most significant change in community care since its introduction in 1993. Under the Community Care Direct Payments Act 1996, local authorities can, instead of providing services themselves, pay money directly to the individual so that they can buy the services they need. Or the person can opt for a mix of services and direct payments. The White Paper *Modernising Social Services* says that direct payments will be available to people of all ages, not just those under 66 as at present. (At the time of writing, this was expected to have come in by the end of 1999.) The Government want 'many more people' to use the direct payments and to have 'real control over how their care needs are provided for'.

A direct payment is not extra income – it must be used to arrange services to meet assessed community care needs, including short periods of respite care. But it is up to the recipient to decide how their needs are met, by whom and when. Direct payments are not taxed or taken into account when assessing income for Social Security benefits.

The advantages of direct payments are obvious. Someone needing help getting out of bed in the morning, for example, may find that the home care assistant employed by the local authority cannot come at the time they want. With direct payments, however, they can arrange for someone else to come at whatever times they want. This can be done either by employing care staff directly or by using a home care agency of the person's choice. The recipient of the direct payment can specify what they want done, how and when, with direct reporting to the recipient.

The local authority should offer direct payments to anybody who meets the national eligibility criteria and who they are satisfied is able and willing to manage them, with – and this is an important point for carers – help if necessary. The criteria for receiving direct payments mainly limit access by people with mental health problems, on probation or with a drug addiction. Most people with arthritis should be eligible to receive them.

Anybody currently receiving community care services, or for whom the local authority decides to arrange community care services, may be entitled to direct payments instead. By January 1999 only 54 out of the 149 councils with responsibility for social services in England and Wales had set up such a system, but with Government encouragement this looks set to increase.

Arranging care through direct payments may sound daunting but why shouldn't people with care needs do what millions of working people do already – arrange domestic help with a third party? Similar schemes in Germany have over a million participants. The local authority should have a support service that can answer queries, and invaluable information and advice can be obtained from the National Centre for Independent Living. Direct payments put the recipient in control – not the local authority and not the carer – and that is what most people with arthritis want.

Penny

'We've a direct payments users' group, which is a source of mutual support and advice, and the local authority has an independent living co-ordinator who works with us. I employ three PAs, and the paperwork – National Insurance, tax, public liability insurance – takes just an hour a week. Less now that I have a computer package to help.'

Independent Living (1993) Fund

People receiving substantial help from their local authority may have access to the Independent Living (1993) Fund. This is a trust financed by the government but administered by seven independent trustees to provide cash payments to severely disabled people under the age of 66. It helps people to live at home rather than in residential care by helping them to meet the additional costs of their domestic or personal care.

The Fund works in partnership with local authorities to enable jointly financed packages of care to be arranged. At the time of writing, if a local authority is providing services and/or direct payments to a minimum value of £200 net a week, the Fund can consider making cash payments of up to £300 a week directly to the disabled person. This must be used to employ people as care assistants. It is not for aids or adaptations, bills or other costs. The primary responsibility for care needs remains with the local authority.

Access to the Independent Living (1993) Fund doesn't depend on a person's National Insurance contributions although account will be taken of their income. It is not available to anyone who has savings of more than £8,000.

For more *i*nformation

ⓘ Age Concern Factsheet 32 *Disability and ageing: your rights to social services.*

ⓘ Age Concern Factsheet 41 *Local authority assessment for community care services.*

ⓘ For more information on direct payments, get the *Guide to Receiving Direct Payments* (code DPG/E), a free introductory guide from the Department of Health (address on p 152).

ⓘ For more information on independent living, contact the National Centre for Independent Living (address on p 156), which can direct you to your local Centre. It can also provide further information on direct payments.

Family

If you are caring for a relative, do not feel obliged to take all responsibility for caring on yourself. Other members of the family can lend a hand, even if you are the closest relative. Think broadly. Even people who live a long way away can provide occasional help – a break away for you or the person for whom you are caring, for example.

Together, make a list of all the tasks that need attention and of everyone who can help. The list you both made for a social services assessment would be a good start but it will be useful to go into even more detail. It's easier to encourage people to help when the tasks are small – they can see that they will be able to cope.

To build support for the arrangements, the best bet is to try to get people to volunteer for particular tasks. People with cars can help with shopping or going out. Younger members of the family can pop in on the way from school or college. Working people might prefer to help financially rather than practically, by paying for a particular service or household aid. They will feel much more comfortable about doing this if they can see that everyone else is doing their bit. Whatever is going to be done, encourage the family member to discuss it with their relative who will be on the receiving end.

Voluntary organisations

The two obvious places you can turn to are carers' organisations and organisations for people with arthritis. Arthritis Care is the UK's leading voluntary organisation for people with arthritis, and can supply the names and addresses of the organisations that deal with specific types of arthritis. The leading carers' organisation is the Carers National Association, which have 120 groups across the country. These provide information, advice and support as well as a voice for carers.

Caroline

'It was the counsellor I saw when I was depressed who first pointed out that I was a full-time carer as well as a full-time worker. It was the first time I'd heard the word. She suggested I go to a meeting with other carers, and I became quite involved. It helped put my own problems in perspective, and at various times I think we all broke down in

95

front of each other. That gave us strength. After my husband Jeff died, I took up campaigning for carers with the local authority and also nationally. Finding a network of people is very important. I didn't realise at first just how important. I don't know if I would have got by without that bedrock, and I also made some strong friendships which I still maintain.'

There are also many local carers' groups or there may be a carers' centre in the area funded by a charity such as The Princess Royal Trust for Carers (address on p 157) or by the local health or social services. Some day centres or family doctor's practices have carers' groups attached to them too. Look up 'carer' in the local phone book, the Internet or ask at the local library, Citizens Advice Bureau or social services office. Many voluntary organisations, including Age Concern and Arthritis Care, come together in the umbrella organisation Carers Alliance.

For more *i*nformation

Contact the various organisations mentioned for further information on how they can help. Their addresses are in the 'Useful addresses' section at the back of this book.

Paid care assistants

There are private agencies that can provide qualified nurses or care assistants. The UK Home Care Association (UKHCA) is a professional body for agencies providing care at home (address on p 159). It can tell you of any members in your area. Or look under 'Nurses' Agencies' in *Yellow Pages*. The advantages of an agency are that it should provide fully refereed staff with back-up in the event of sickness. It will also deal with tax and National Insurance. But it will probably be more expensive than recruiting someone yourself.

Bringing a professional into a personal relationship can sometimes have its problems, as Diane found. She has had arthritis since she was 18 months old, and one of her carers is her mother.

Diane

'It's difficult to get the balance. She's my mother but I'm an adult. With a paid carer you can state what you want and how you want it done. You can't do that with your mum.

'It was difficult when I first employed a personal assistant. My mum felt she was being pushed out. But we're open and we talk about things. Although parents can be over-protective of disabled children, my mum respects me as a person with my own opinions. I involved her in the interviewing for my personal assistant, which I think helped. It's meant that we've both got time and space away from each other. Now, I'm very close to my mum. We have a nice relationship.'

To find someone yourself, simply advertise in the local paper or JobCentre. The national magazines *The Lady* and *Choice* are also widely used for this sort of advertising. Think carefully about what you actually need. Is it a qualified nurse or just someone who'll be there when needed? Penny has had about seven personal assistants (PAs) over the years.

Penny

'Finding the right PA is very important; they need to understand the distinction between a PA and a carer. The main thing is to be clear about what you want. You need to find the right place to advertise for a PA or go to an agency. I use *The Big Issue* and the local paper.

'I chat to people for quite a long time and I'm fairly up front about what I want. Being clear about what is needed is vital and that's why I provide a list of exactly what needs to be done. I want to put off people who aren't suitable and I interview only the two or three who seem most appropriate. For me, feeling they'll fit into my life is more important than experience. I have interviewed people who have no experience and are worried about that. I'm not. If someone hasn't done it before, they'll do it my way. Our independent living group has designed an application form that I use. Most local schemes will have one. Timing is important, too. The summer is never very good for recruiting.

'If you are worried about interviewing prospective PAs, get a friend or an advocate or someone from your local independent living group to help. It's not as hard as you might think.'

If you do the recruiting yourself, check out references and be prepared to take on the responsibilities of an employer – including a contract of terms and conditions, statutory sick pay, National Insurance contributions, income tax and insurance. Needless to say, discuss it all with the person who will be receiving the care, regardless of who is actually doing the hiring.

For more *i*nformation

❶ For information about hiring someone yourself, get the *Personal Assistants Employer's Handbook*, published by the West of England Centre for Independent Living (address on p 160).

❶ The Disablement Income Group produce a booklet *Recruiting and Employing a Personal Care Worker.*

❶ The National Centre for Independent Living (address on p 156) can also provide further information on employing personal assistants.

5 Planning for change

It is all very well reading about the things discussed in this book but at some point you and the person you are caring for will have to act on some of them. You will certainly have to plan for them. But how do you do that?

It is easy to say that it's the decision of the person with arthritis but it's never as simple as that. Making a decision is difficult. And once it's made, expressing it can be even harder. This chapter looks at how you can talk together to try to ensure that, as far as possible, what happens to them is what the person with arthritis wants.

Jack

'It's easy to say "Talk about it" but you have to make sure that it actually happens and that you talk properly. Turn off the telly, turn off the radio and sit down together.'

You will need to be open minded. This may mean challenging some of your own views about the right and wrong way to live. Try asking questions rather than giving what you think are the answers. When discussing the way forward for you both, it is important that each of you feels able to be honest about what you want. Although the person you are caring for should make decisions about their

99

life, your life is equally important and there should be room for give and take on both sides.

Important discussions such as these can be exhausting, so aim to take a break after an hour and a half. And don't aim to resolve everything in one session. You may find that you will both want to mull over what each other has said and come back to the subject some days later.

Three key questions

Few problems are straightforward and, when it comes to caring, it is probably fair to say that none of them is. Everything is related to something else, and it can be difficult to know where to start talking. But there are three key questions to keep in your mind, however complicated the discussion gets:

- Where is the person with arthritis now? (the current situation)
- Where do they want to be? (the preferred situation)
- How do they get there? (the route)

The attitudes with which you embark on these discussions will make a big difference to how you both feel about them and their outcomes. You will need to show the person you are caring for and their views:

- **respect** – which involves accepting their concerns, however unfounded they may seem, giving them your full attention, time and effort, and letting them know that you believe they are capable of making their own decisions;
- **empathy** – trying to understand how they feel, not deciding how you think they ought to feel or projecting onto them how you might feel in a similar situation;
- **genuineness** – meaning what you say and saying what you mean in a tactful but not a defensive, emotional or manipulative way.

How to listen effectively

Body language does make a difference. Remember SOLER:

S face the other person **S**quarely;

O sit **O**penly without crossed arms and legs;

L **L**ean towards the other attentively;

E maintain **E**ye contact;

R be **R**elaxed.

All this can help you to encourage the person you are caring for to speak frankly. You will certainly want to think about the ways of listening that promote communication:

- **active** – listening, nodding and giving verbal encouragement to go on;
- **attentive** – not interrupting but maintaining encouraging eye contact;
- **reflecting** – bouncing back something that has been said to encourage more and to check that you have understood;
- **paraphrasing** – summarising what has just been said, to make sure that you really understand what is being said and how the person feels about it.

You will want to ask questions. Indeed, you will need to ask questions. But ask only one at a time. Multiple questions – Have you X; what about Y; do you want Z? – are confusing. And avoid asking leading questions of the variety 'Wouldn't it be great if you did this?'

Closed questions (ones to which the answer is 'Yes' or 'No') are best to ascertain matters of fact. Open questions (such as 'What do you think about that?') are better for drawing out feelings. Try to be gently probing rather than blunt. 'Why did you do that?' can sound threatening and prompt a defensive response. 'How did you feel about what happened?' is much warmer.

The person you are talking to will have their own prejudices just like everyone else, and these may be getting in the way of their making a decision. For example, misconceptions about what sheltered housing actually is might prevent its being considered. Sometimes ignorance may be the problem. For example, not claiming a benefit because the person doesn't know it exists. You need to address these by challenging – again gently. 'What do you think stops you from doing Z?' or 'What do you think about Y?'

Even in the example of the unclaimed benefit, a tentative approach is best. Don't say 'You should claim housing benefit'. Letting the person with arthritis make the decision for themselves isn't just about showing respect, it's practical from your point of view too. The person will be much more committed to the idea if they come to it themselves.

Setting goals

What we want is rarely as simple as deciding whether to have tea or coffee with our breakfast. We normally work within a hazy framework of vague aspirations and unstated intentions. Distilling these into clear goals will help you both a lot. It's easy to say what these goals might be in general terms – staying in my own home, reducing my medication, taking more exercise – but clear goals may only emerge after going around a lot of conversational houses.

Goals should be:

- **Specific** Words such as 'better' aren't helpful. If the goal is to lose weight, how much weight? This makes it far easier to know whether (or when) the goal has been achieved.
- **Attainable** Achievable short-term targets are better than pie-in-the-sky long-term ideals. To have more money might be a desirable goal but, if someone is claiming all the benefits they are entitled to and cannot work, it may not be achievable. Breaking up a major task into small, attainable, chunks can really help here.
- **Relevant** The goal has to be something the person wants to achieve – not a goal imposed from outside – and one that really will take them closer to where they want to be.

List all the possible goals and assess each on its merits as seen by the person with arthritis before choosing one or two to focus on.

Taking action

Question three – how to get there? – is the tough one but you don't need to know the answers. You just need to know the questions. Between you, think of all the possible ways of achieving the goal, however ridiculous they may seem. This is sometimes called brainstorming. You'll probably have a laugh doing it and come up with a longish list for even the most impossible-seeming idea. Assess all the options. If there truly isn't a route to the desired goal, you might have to reconsider question two – where does the person want to be? The conversation may go back and forth here.

Once a route is identified, you might want to think about an action plan. What needs to be done and in what order? By whom? By when? What information do you need? What problems might arise and how might they be overcome?

The three-question approach is flexible and will work with virtually any situation, from a simple one such as whether to buy a back-support cushion to a complex one such as where to live. Sometimes it will work very informally; on other occasions it might make sense to write down your lists of ideas and actions. The approach works on a number of levels. On the way to one major goal – living independently in my own home – there may be a number of intermediate goals, such as getting a local authority assessment, claiming all my benefits, getting the bathroom altered and so on. It can help whenever there is difference between what is and what is desired.

Asking the three key questions is not original. If you go for counselling – and many people with arthritis and those caring for them benefit from it – you will probably find that they use a similar approach. And don't be surprised if you find the person you are caring for trying it out on you.

Fiona

'I didn't just come straight out and tell my mother I was getting a professional carer. I talked to her about the problems my needs were causing for her in running her own life. Her relationship with my dad, her relationship with my sister who lives quite a long way away, the fact that her career was on hold – all these came up when we were talking. It wasn't easy at first. She did her usual routine – knocking back her tea saying "Well, I must get on". I moved the conversation on myself I suppose by taking her hand and telling her how much I valued what she did. That got her talking to me seriously. That and the fact that I stuck my wheelchair between her and the kitchen door!'

For more *i*nformation

The British Association for Counselling publishes a directory of counsellors in the UK (address on p 150).

6 What do you need to think about?

The previous chapter considered how you and the person you are caring for might approach problem solving. This chapter looks at some of the specific problems you might need to solve, and offers some of the information and advice that might help you to do that.

Prakash

'It sounds such a simple thing but the turning point was when we just sat down and made a list. We realised that we needed to think about the problems or difficulties that the arthritis had created. Then we could find out the necessary information and work out how to solve them – with help if we needed it.'

Long-term medical prognosis

To make the best caring choices, it is important to get a good idea of how the arthritis is going to develop. A social services assessment will help but ideally you should both discuss the prognosis with the GP or consultant. Doctors can sometimes feel uncomfortable about being put on the spot like this but, if you explain why you are asking, most will try to be helpful. Make sure that the people you are dealing with, particularly social services, know the prognosis. Having the right aids and adaptations in place promptly can reduce joint damage and subsequent loss of mobility.

Rheumatoid arthritis varies considerably in severity. Perhaps a third of people who develop rheumatoid arthritis will only ever have very mild disease. The majority will have periods of remission but also more serious pain, swelling and flares throughout their lives. Possibly 5 per cent develop severe disease with extensive disability but even in this group many people continue to live independently. Initially it may be difficult to tell which category an individual will be in but improved testing is making this easier.

In most cases osteoarthritis will get worse with time but it is generally steady, which makes planning a little easier.

Dealing with crises

In older people, arthritis can come on very suddenly, particularly rheumatoid arthritis. It can be triggered by a crisis. Brenda's came on after a heart operation.

Brenda

'It started in Bognor on holiday. We'd been walking all day and at about midnight I just couldn't breathe. I was rushed into hospital. They did some tests and found I had a leaky heart valve that had to be replaced. I'd always had high blood pressure and high cholesterol. I think the heart problem triggered everything else. The body is like an old car, I suppose – once something goes, everything else starts to pack in.

'The arthritis came on when I was in rehabilitation after the heart operation but I couldn't understand it at first. It was far worse than any pain I'd had before and that includes the night I was rushed to hospital with my heart. One night I woke up and my wrist was aching. It quickly moved to my knee and then to my feet. Blood tests confirmed that I had rheumatoid arthritis. I think it was the shock of the operation or perhaps a reaction to one of the many antibiotics I had afterwards that triggered it.'

In the event of any sudden change in circumstances, including rapid onset of the disease, the local authority can provide emergency services before a full needs assessment has been made. Other typical situations eligible for emergency provision (under section 47 of the NHS and Community Care Act 1990) are a fall or a change in caring arrangements.

Falls are a particular risk for people with arthritis. They are more likely to happen and their impact can be more serious. (Some suggestions for reducing the risks are given on page 130.) In most cases, a person with arthritis who has a fall should have an X-ray to check that there is no damage. Even if nothing is broken, they are likely to stiffen up – which may increase care needs for a few days.

If the person is taken into hospital, make sure you know when they will be discharged. Hospitals should not discharge someone after a fall, for example, without ensuring that any care needs at home will be met. Don't rush into making changes in care or domestic arrangements after a fall but, equally, don't assume that its effects will disappear with the bruises. Confidence is likely to be affected – for many people, a fall becomes symbolic of losing control of one's life. Time and encouragement are the best you can give in these circumstances.

For more *i*nformation

Age Concern Factsheet 37 *Hospital discharge arrangements and NHS continuing health care services.*

Money

Money management

Disability can be expensive. Housing, transport and day-to-day household expenses often cost more when you have arthritis. Many of these costs are reflected in the costs of caring. Even if the person is living independently or in a residential home, you will still probably incur additional transport costs from more frequent visits, higher telephone bills and the cost of any fees, aids or alterations to which you contribute. If someone is living in your home, you will need to think about additional food, heating, transport, living aids and adaptations to your home.

Extra costs of living with arthritis include:

■ additional heating and hot water;
■ personal assistance;
■ domestic help;
■ gardening and household maintenance;
■ home adaptations;
■ special equipment;
■ mobility – car adaptations and taxi fares;
■ special diets;
■ prescription and non-prescription drugs;
■ non-NHS treatment, such as complementary therapies.

It is unlikely that you will need to take over formal responsibility for the finances of someone whose only impairment is arthritis but it is important that both of you know exactly what your income and expenses are. An open relationship about money and clear, transparent practices are important. Most family rows are over money, and a caring relationship might complicate matters still further.

If money is a problem for you, don't be embarrassed about seeking help. Many local authorities have a specialist money advice worker. The Citizens Advice Bureau can also be very helpful. A money adviser will take you through your finances systematically and show you how to maximise income and minimise expenditure. It really can work – especially when you feel that you just cannot make ends meet.

State benefits

This section looks at the benefits available to you both. There are more than you might imagine and, despite everything we hear about fraud, millions of pounds in benefits go unclaimed every week by those entitled to them, particularly among older people.

The ones most commonly unclaimed are Income Support, Council Tax Benefit and Housing Benefit, which is ignored by more than half a million potential claimants.

The information here is as accurate as possible but benefits, rates and the regulations governing them do change. The Benefits Enquiry Line on 0800 88 22 00, which gives confidential advice to disabled or sick people and their carers, will be able to advise you on any changes. Many Citizens Advice Bureaux have a benefits adviser who can advise you both about the benefits to which you are entitled, or try the local welfare rights group or law centre. Neither you nor the person you are caring for should have any qualms about claiming these benefits. That is why you and your family have paid taxes and National Insurance. Remember that carers save the state billions of pounds, and disabled people surely have a right to help.

Benefits that depend on the claimant having paid sufficient National Insurance contributions are known as *contributory*. Those that depend on how much money or savings the person has are known as *means-tested*. Some benefits are taxable although, of course, you will only have to pay tax on them if your total taxable income – including these benefits – exceeds your tax allowance.

This section is divided into four parts:

- benefits for the person with arthritis;
- benefits for the carer;
- benefits for people with a state pension;
- benefits for people on low incomes.

Benefits for the person with arthritis

There are many benefits that can be claimed by a sick or disabled person. The Benefits Agency have pamphlets and application forms, which will give full details. There is only room in this book to consider some of the main ones that may be relevant to you and the person you are caring for.

109

Attendance Allowance

Attendance Allowance is a tax-free, non-contributory, non-means-tested benefit for people over 65 who need help with personal care or need someone to watch over them because of physical or mental illness or disability. These needs must normally have existed for at least six months. The allowance does not have to be used to pay for care, but the local authority can take it into account when assessing whether and how much a person should pay for any social services they receive.

There is a higher and a lower rate. The *lower rate* is paid if the person needs frequent help throughout the day or at least twice at night. The *higher rate* is paid if the person needs such help during the day *and* at night.

Disability Living Allowance

Like Attendance Allowance, this is a tax-free, non-contributory, non-means-tested benefit. The person will have become disabled and made a claim before the age of 65 because they need help with personal care or getting around, or both. Normally, these needs must have existed for three months and be expected to continue for at least another three months. There are two components: the care component and the mobility component.

The **care component** is for people needing personal care (eg help with washing, dressing or cooking). It is paid at three rates, according to the amount of care required:

- the *higher rate* if help is needed both day and night;
- the *middle rate* if help is needed day or night;
- the *lower rate* if some help is needed during some of the day.

Payment of the benefit may stop if the claimant moves into a residential care or nursing home. They should not be worse off after contributing to their home fees.

Recipients of the higher rate are automatically classified as 80 per cent disabled for Severe Disablement Allowance.

The **mobility component** is for people who need help getting around. This is paid at two rates: higher and lower.

The *higher rate* is paid to a number of categories of people. The relevant category for someone with arthritis is that of people who cannot walk at all or are virtually unable to walk. People receiving this higher rate may be exempt from road tax (contact the DLA Unit of the Department of Social Security (address on p 160, under 'Vehicle Excise Duty') for information); they will qualify for the Orange Badge scheme (Blue Badge from 2000) but anyone claiming since April 1997 is no longer deemed automatically to satisfy the Severe Disablement Allowance 80 per cent disability test. If the award is made for three years or more, they may be able to get a car or electric wheelchair under the Motability scheme. Apply immediately – it is not necessary to wait the three years implied in the regulations.

The *lower rate* is payable if a claimant can walk but is unable to do so out of doors unless someone is with them.

The mobility component of the Disability Living Allowance is not affected by moving into a residential care home or nursing home.

To claim, the person completes form DLA1, which includes a section for the claimant's own assessment of how their illness or disability affects them. (The form is quite long but do not be put off by this: the Disability Alliance (address on p 152) has a guide on completing it – *The DLA Checklist* – which you may find helpful.) In some cases a medical examination will be arranged to obtain further information. Claimants who do not want to fill in the self-assessment section can ask for a medical examination instead or can ask for someone from the Benefits Agency to visit. New claims and some reviews are dealt with at Disability Benefit Centres.

Payment of Disability Living Allowance may be combined with other benefits so that they are all paid together.

Severe disability premium

This may be payable to a disabled person who lives alone and receives Attendance Allowance or the middle or higher level of the care component of the Disability Living Allowance and no one is receiving Invalid Care Allowance for looking after them. It may also be payable to someone living with a partner who also receives Attendance Allowance. The rules are complicated, so it is best to seek advice before claiming this premium.

Statutory Sick Pay

An employee who has to take time off sick with arthritis is entitled to Statutory Sick Pay, just like any other member of staff. This includes most people (employees) who pay Class 1 National Insurance contributions. It is paid for up to 28 weeks, after which Incapacity Benefit must be claimed. If the employee returns to work for less than eight weeks and then is off sick again, it counts, for the purposes of Statutory Sick Pay, as a single spell of illness.

Incapacity Benefit

Incapacity Benefit is for people under state pension age who cannot work because of illness or disability. It cannot be claimed by anyone who was over the state pension age when their illness began. It is paid at three rates:

- at the *short-term lower rate* for the first 28 weeks of illness, to people who are self-employed, unemployed, non-employed or employed but not eligible for Statutory Sick Pay;
- at the *short-term higher rate* from week 29 to week 52 of their illness to all the above plus employees who have received Statutory Sick Pay;
- at the *long-term rate* to all the above from week 53 of their illness.

An important exception here concerns people receiving Disability Living Allowance (discussed above). People claiming the care component of Disability Living Allowance at the highest rate are entitled to the long-term rate of Incapacity Benefit from week 29 of their illness rather than from week 53. This also applies to people who are terminally ill.

For the first 28 weeks, a doctor's certificate of inability to work should be sufficient. After that, the claimant may well have to fill in a questionnaire from the Benefits Agency and be examined by one of their doctors. This is called the 'all work test' and has been very controversial, especially with people with arthritis. The fact that the disease is widely misunderstood may count against people with arthritis. A claimant won't have to go through the work test if they have already been found to be 80 per cent disabled under the regulations for Severe Disablement Allowance.

A claimant can appeal if they are told they are fit for work. Appeals go to a Disability Appeals Tribunal. More appeals are successful than you might imagine.

People receiving Incapacity Benefit are allowed to do voluntary work without this affecting their benefits. With the agreement of the Benefits Agency, they may receive what are called therapeutic earnings – payment for work that the doctor considers will help improve or prevent the deterioration of the claimant's medical condition: no more than 16 hours per week paying no more than a set limit per week.

Changes to Incapacity Benefit are planned for 2001/2002. The Government intends to tighten the contribution conditions and to reduce the amount of benefit paid to people with private pensions over a certain amount.

Severe Disablement Allowance

Severe Disablement Allowance is for people aged 16 and over who qualify before reaching the age of 65 and who have been unable to work for 28 weeks but are not eligible for Incapacity Benefit because they have not paid enough National Insurance contributions. Similar additions apply as for Incapacity Benefit (above), and there are the same regulations for voluntary work and therapeutic earnings.

The Government is planning to abolish Severe Disablement Allowance for new claimants from 2001/2002. People disabled from a young age will be able to claim Incapacity Benefit.

Recipients must be 80 per cent disabled. People receiving the higher rate of the care component of the Disability Living Allowance (see earlier) are automatically so classified. So are people who are blind or who have already been as assessed as 80 per cent disabled for an Industrial Injuries Disablement Benefit or War Disablement Pension. Others will have to have a medical examination.

Disabled Person's Tax Credit

In October 1999, Disability Working Allowance was replaced by Disabled Person's Tax Credit, which is more generous.

People with a disability that puts them at a disadvantage in the job market and are receiving certain benefits, such as Disability Living Allowance or Attendance Allowance, and are working at least 16 hours per week may get the tax credit from the Inland Revenue. Whether a person qualifies and, if so, the level of the credit depends on their earnings and whether they are married (or living together as though married), single or have children.

A person's savings (and that of their partner) are taken into account:

■ anyone with savings or capital over £16,000 will not be eligible;
■ someone with savings or capital between £3,000 and £16,000 will receive tax credit according to the amount they have.

Many working people with arthritis will be eligible. The Disabled Person's Tax Credit Helpline (0845 605 5858) can give advice about this new scheme and how to apply for it.

Benefits for carers

There is only room in this book to consider some of the more obvious state benefits. The Benefits Agency should give you full details.

Invalid Care Allowance

This is a non-contributory, non-means-tested, taxable, weekly benefit for people of working age who are giving 'regular and substantial' care at least 35 hours a week to a severely disabled person who is receiving Attendance Allowance or Disability Living Allowance at the highest or middle rate of the care component. The Benefits Agency advises not to delay making a claim for Invalid Care Allowance because you are waiting to hear if the person you are caring for is eligible for the Disability Living Allowance.

Invalid Care Allowance cannot be claimed by someone who is in full-time education (21 hours or more a week) or who earns more than £50 a week after deducting allowable expenses. If another Social Security benefit such as the retirement pension is being claimed and the amount received is less than the Invalid Care Allowance, the difference can be made up to the weekly rate for that Allowance. If another Social Security benefit such as the widow's pension is being claimed and the amount received is higher than the Invalid Care Allowance, that Allowance is not paid (although Class 1 National Insurance contributions will be). Additional Invalid Care Allowance is paid to carers with dependent children.

Invalid Care Allowance may affect both the carer's and the disabled person's entitlement to, and rates of, Income Support or JobSeeker's Allowance. A disabled person cannot claim the severe disability premium under Income Support if their carer is claiming Invalid Care Allowance. However, the carer will qualify for a carer's premium if they claim Income Support or related benefit such as Housing Benefit or Council Tax Benefit. This premium entitlement exists even when Invalid Care Allowance is not being paid because the carer is receiving an overlapping benefit (such as the widow's pension mentioned in the example above).

The Allowance continues to be paid if the carer takes a break – up to a total of 12 weeks in any six-month period, though no more than four of these can be holiday weeks. Payment of the Allowance also continues if the disabled person goes into hospital, but stops if they cease to receive Disability Living Allowance or Attendance Allowance.

Warning If the person you care for receives the severe disability premium, they will lose it if you are awarded Invalid Care Allowance. You might be eligible for the carer's premium (£13.95 in 1999) but the severe disability premium is worth more (£39.75 in 1999). If you are not sure whether to claim Invalid Care Allowance, get advice first.

Home Responsibilities Protection

If you are looking after a disabled person and cannot work or do not pay enough National Insurance contributions to count for retirement pension purposes, you may be entitled to Home Responsibilities Protection. This protects your right to a state pension and, in the case of a man, his widow's right to widow's benefits.

Home Responsibilities Protection reduces the number of qualifying years needed for a basic pension at the standard rate. The minimum number of years to which it can be reduced is 20. It is available for complete tax years in which you have been caring for someone but are not entitled to Invalid Care Allowance. The Benefits Agency leaflet CF411 explains the system in more detail and includes an application form.

Benefits for people with a state pension

Benefits that can be claimed by someone already receiving a state pension include Attendance Allowance, Christmas Bonus, Council Tax Benefit, Disability Living Allowance, Housing Benefit, Income Support, help with NHS costs, Over-80s Pension Category D, War Disablement Pension, War Pensioner's Mobility Supplement, War Widow's Pension, Widow's Pension and Winter Fuel Payments. The Benefits Agency should give you full details.

Benefits for people on low incomes

The benefits that can be claimed by people on low incomes include Council Tax Benefit, Disability Working Allowance, Family Credit, Housing Benefit, Income Support, JobSeeker's Allowance, help with NHS costs and access to Work Incentive Schemes. The Benefits Agency should give you full details.

Depending on your exact circumstances, you might want to explore your own entitlement and that of the person for whom you are caring to the following.

Income Support This is payable if you are on a low income and working less than 16 hours a week. It is also a passport to other benefits, such as community care grants, Cold Weather Payments, Housing Benefit, and free NHS prescriptions, sight tests and dental treatment.

Family Credit This is payable if you have a family and are on a low income but work more than 16 hours a week.

Housing Benefit and **Council Tax Benefit** These are payable by the local authority to people on low incomes who need help to pay their rent or council tax.

Tips on claiming benefits

- ■ If in doubt, claim. The Citizens Advice Bureau or the Carers National Association CarersLine can do a benefits check for you to make sure you are not overlooking anything.
- ■ Be honest about what you are unable to do. Put simply, if you cannot do something as often as you want, you *cannot* do it even if you can do it occasionally or only need a little help.
- ■ With benefits that include premiums, make sure that you are getting all you are entitled to.
- ■ If you are going to claim a disability benefit, you may wish to get advice first from a local disability group or call Arthritis Care's information line. Talk to them again if you are turned down and plan to appeal.

■ *How to Appeal*, Benefits Agency leaflet N1246, outlines the appeals procedure. Copies can be obtained from your local Benefits Agency office.

Pensions

You are entitled to a state retirement pension when you reach state pension age – currently 60 for a woman, 65 for a man – if you have paid or been credited with enough National Insurance contributions. The state retirement pension is taxable.

The basic state retirement pension is the same for men, for women who have paid their own standard rate National Insurance and for widows who claim on their deceased husband's contributions. Married women who are not entitled on the basis of their own National Insurance contributions may receive a pension on the basis of their husband's. A man who became a widower before the age of 65 who is not entitled to a full basic pension can have his wife's contributions taken into account to give him a higher pension. There are a number of factors that can increase your state retirement pension: increments, earnings-related additions, having dependent children, supporting another adult, being over 80 and, in certain cases, an Invalidity Allowance. The first two of these are outlined below.

Increments You can increase your state retirement pension if you put off receiving it for up to five years after state pension age and do not claim an excluding benefit. Two benefits that come into this category are Severe Disablement Allowance and Invalid Care Allowance: days for which these (or any of the other 'excluding benefits') have been received are excluded from the calculation for an increment. A woman can earn increments over the age of 65 on a married woman's pension if her husband is deferring his pension.

Earnings-related additions These may be payable to people who paid employee National Insurance contributions between 1961 and 1975 (called graduated retirement benefit) and to those who paid standard rate employee National Insurance after 5 April 1978 (called state earnings-related pension scheme or SERPS).

People receiving the state retirement pension can claim other benefits, including Income Support. Everyone over 60 is entitled to free NHS prescriptions and may get help with other health costs. The Government have said that all pensioners should have a minimum income of £78 a week. They are also keen to encourage pensioners to claim Income Support; they estimate that up to 700,000 pensioners who are eligible do not claim it.

A widow is entitled to benefits if her husband paid sufficient National Insurance contributions. These include the Widow's Payment on death, the Widow's Pension (currently paid to childless widows over 45) and the Widowed Mother's Allowance (currently paid to widows of any age with dependent children). Major changes are planned for widow's benefits.

You and/or the person you care for may be entitled to an occupational pension. If you have paid into one, your employer should provide you with the relevant information. Seek advice if you are dissatisfied or concerned. If necessary, you can involve the Occupational Pensions Regulatory Authority. You may also have a personal pension. Any problems here that an independent financial adviser cannot resolve satisfactorily should be taken to the Financial Services Authority.

Insurance

Check your entitlement to help under any insurance policies you or the person you are caring for might have. If you have private medical insurance, don't assume that you will be covered. Insurance companies don't like paying out, and when you are talking about a long-term condition such as arthritis they are very reluctant. Check the small print.

The Disability Discrimination Act 1995 makes it unlawful to discriminate against disabled people in connection with the provision of goods, facilities and services. This includes insurance. However, the Act (and subsequent Regulations) states that there are circumstances in which insurers may differentiate between disabled and non-disabled people. This means that insurance companies need to be able to account for any difference in their treatment of disabled and non-disabled people, and this must be based on reliable information relevant to the risk being insured. When insurers use eligibility criteria – for example, age and employment status – these criteria cannot be based on disability but can exclude claims arising out of the disability. This exclusion must be 'fair' – that is, based on evidence and not assumptions.

For more *i*nformation

i For information on benefits, contact the Benefits Enquiry Line on 0800 88 22 00, a local advice bureau or disability organisation. The Benefits Agency also has a good website on the Internet, with lots of information on individual benefits.

i A good introductory leaflet is the Benefits Agency's *Sick or Disabled* (leaflet SD1), available from the post office or from the local Benefits Agency office.

i *The DLA Checklist* is a guide produced by the Disability Alliance (address on p 152) to help in completing the application for Disability Living Allowance.

i *Your Rights* by Sally West, published annually by Age Concern England.

i Age Concern has a number of factsheets that may be of help. For example:

- Factsheet 17 *Housing Benefit and Council Tax Benefit;*

- Factsheet 18 *A brief guide to money benefits;*

- Factsheet 20 *National Insurance contributions and qualifying for a pension;*

- Factsheet 21 *The Council Tax and older people;*

- Factsheet 25 *Income Support and the Social Fund;*

- Factsheet 34 *Attendance Allowance and Disability Living Allowance.*

Aids and adaptations

Four main types of equipment are available:

- An item or gadget designed specifically for disabled people to overcome a particular difficulty (eg a wheelchair, bath board, raised toilet seat or orthopaedic footwear).
- Standard equipment with a particularly helpful feature that takes the physical effort out of the activity (eg an electric tin opener, a food processor, a computer, Velcro fastenings or power steering on a car).
- Standard equipment that has been adapted (eg a tap with a long handle, a comb with a long handle).
- A 'custom made' item to suit a particular individual's need. These can be made at home, commercially or by the voluntary organisation REMAP.

Below are some examples of the types of aids that may be particularly useful for a person with arthritis:

- People with weak or painful hands often prefer lightweight gadgets or appliances with larger, easy-to-grip controls or handles that require less force. Rubber knob turners can change fiddly controls into easy ones. A person with arthritis might also benefit from a gadget being secured in place so that one hand is not needed to hold or steady it – a slicing guide for bread, for example.
- People using wheelchairs will need sufficient space for turning and transferring. They need appliances that are positioned so they can be operated within their reach from the chair and with sufficient knee room to get in close. Cooker controls must be at the front of the cooker, for example.
- People who find it difficult to bend may need long-handled equipment – grabbers, reachers or pick-up sticks. Gadgets need to be positioned above waist height, including, for example, electric socket extenders. Raised seats may be helpful, but this need not mean buying new furniture – specially designed wooden blocks can do the job. The legs need to fit snugly into

the raised blocks; simply resting them on a brick or something similar could be dangerous.

■ Most people with arthritis will want appliances that aren't tiring to use. This includes labour-saving devices such as washing machines, electric wheelchairs and food processors as well as smaller gadgets such as teapot pourers.

Clothing is a good example of how a little ingenuity goes a long way. With such a variety of fabrics, fastenings and styles to choose from, it is usually possible to find something you feel good wearing and that you can actually get into. And think laterally. Why struggle with a tie when you can buy a clip-on? If you can't get a good loose fit in your size, buy larger sizes. Women could check out the larger, baggier sizes in the men's department.

Bigger buttons are easier than smaller ones. A big tab on a zip makes it easier to move – attaching a cord can also help. Velcro, with its hundreds of tiny fibre hooks, is easy to use. Accessible fastenings also help – front rather than back fastenings on bras, for example. Many popular items of clothing need no fastening at all, including jogging suits, tracksuits, shawls, wrap-around skirts and kimonos.

What do people with arthritis need?

A survey by the British League Against Rheumatism in 1994 found the following levels of demand for specialist equipment among people with arthritis:

55%	bath seat/shower stool
55%	raised toilet seat
43%	shower
40%	bath/toilet rails
26%	entrance rails
25%	chair adaptation
18%	extra stair rail
15%	help alert system
14%	stair or other lift

There are four ways to get hold of aids and equipment:

■ through the occupational therapist from the health authority or social services;
■ buying them privately;
■ from charities or other organisations;
■ making them.

Getting equipment through the health or local authority

The health authority has an obligation to provide sick and disabled people with the medical support aids and equipment they need. The local authority, as discussed in Chapter 4, can provide non-medical support aids and equipment – they have an obligation to assess someone's need for these but not necessarily to respond to it. Inevitably, this gives rise to a number of grey areas over exactly what is 'medical' and neither authority will willingly pay for something that might not be their responsibility. Persevere.

Some of the medical items that will help someone with arthritis live at home can be prescribed by the GP – support bandages, for example – but most will require a referral. Physiotherapists can provide walking aids. Both physiotherapists and chiropodists may be able to help with footwear. A hospital foot specialist such as an orthotist or podiatrist certainly can. District nurses can help with equipment for the bathroom (raised toilet seats, bath rails and so on) and bedroom (bed hoists, raised beds and the like). Consultants may be able to help with special medical equipment. Medical and nursing products provided by the health authority may incur a small charge.

Wheelchairs are usually provided through the NHS wheelchair service, which is able to provide a wide range of wheelchairs and cushions. Alternatively, they can give a voucher towards the person with arthritis buying one themselves.

Local authority social services departments have responsibility for the aids needed for washing, eating, dressing or going to the toilet, so you can see where the overlap can occur. They can also help with grab rails and disabled parking spaces. See the section on page 87 for how to approach social services.

In some cases the Disability Support Team (DST) at the Employment Service can provide special equipment that a disabled person might need to do their job. For example, I have a repetitive strain injury, which makes computer keyboard work very difficult. The DST provided a computer powerful enough to run software enabling me to dictate into the computer rather than type. The local JobCentre can provide further information on services for disabled workers.

Make sure that your GP is aware of any problems you have accessing statutory services, as a doctor or social worker's referral may get things moving.

Caroline

'Be honest with your GP about your problems. Don't kid yourself that you can cope. Ask politely for what you want. Don't wait to be asked or for it to be offered. Outline the difficulty clearly and say you want professional help to deal with it.

'I can't fault social services, but I knew the channels to go down. I made sure I knew everybody's name. They put in handrails, a bath unit, a special chair and offered a stairlift. Community care should be about outcomes not systems, and the outcomes should be based on the needs of the users. It must also be recognised that the needs of carers and of users are different. They will only come to understand this if we keep telling them.'

Buying equipment

With our growing older population, there is an expanding market for specialist aids and gadgets from jar openers and key turners to wheelchairs and stairlifts. You can find your local stores in the *Yellow Pages* under 'Disabled Equipment', and most pharmacist/

chemist shops have a catalogue of equipment for people with disabilities. Do shop around, though. Many of the products and catalogues targeted specifically at disabled people are not good value for money. Some items are available more cheaply through mainstream outlets; others are simply not a lot of good. Discuss any possible purchase – particularly a larger one – with a health professional. Will it really help? It is possible to spend a lot of money on a product that is not really suitable.

A good retailer should allow you to try out a product either in the store or at home. Some stores may hire equipment. Better still is a visit to a Disabled Living Centre. Here you should be able to view and assess equipment with the benefit of an occupational therapist's advice and without the attentions of a shopkeeper. There are about 40 Disabled Living Centres across the UK. For the address of the one nearest you, contact the Disabled Living Centres Council. Another possibility may be Naidex, a company that runs exhibitions around the country at which manufacturers show their wares.

Finally, try your library or local disability group for books that list aids and adaptations. Two good ones are listed on page 127 under 'For more information', which also mentions the factsheets from the Disabled Living Foundation.

Help paying for aids

Some financial help may be available for buying an item. The government Social Fund can give community care grants to people receiving Income Support. Your local Benefits Agency will give you an application form, and Arthritis Care, a local disability organisation, welfare rights group or Citizens Advice Bureau may be able to give you some advice about completing it.

Some charities can also help with payment. Check a book called *A Guide to Grants for Individuals in Need* published by the Directory of Social Change. It should be in your local library. Most charities will want applications to be made through, or at least countersigned by, a social worker or health professional.

VAT is not charged on support aids and equipment provided that they are for the use of a disabled person. You will have to sign a declaration to that effect. Contact the local Customs and Excise office and ask for VAT notice 7017 on VAT exemption, which includes a copy of the declaration form.

Equipment from charities

Some charities may also be able to help with the provision of equipment, either short term or long term. The British Red Cross, for example, lend basic items, including wheelchairs. Some charities may make a small charge.

Creative thinking

The more inventive prefer to make aids themselves. A visit to a Disabled Living Centre or disability aids shop can be a good source of inspiration.

In many cases, solving a problem may well be simpler than having an adaptation made to the house or even buying a gadget. Changing the way something is done may be all that is needed. If it is difficult to get in and out of the bath, a shower may be easier. If cooking is difficult or tiring, what about the possibilities offered by modern technology – the microwave, freezer and slow cooker, for example? If the difficulty is ironing, how about buying clothes that can be drip-dried?

It can be tough to change an activity that you have been doing in the same way for years – it can feel like a threat to your independence, even your whole being. But if it results in an approach that is quicker, easier and less tiring, it must be worth considering.

For more *i*nformation

- The Disabled Living Foundation is an invaluable source of information on equipment. They produce factsheets on every type of device you can think of and more, and also have a helpline (0870 603 9177).

ℹ For more on finding aids and adaptations, contact the Disabled Living Centres Council and the Disabled Living Foundation (addresses on p 153).

ℹ For further details about custom-made equipment, contact REMAP GB (address on p 158).

ℹ Age Concern Factsheet 42 *Disability equipment and how to get it.*

ℹ *Getting Equipment for Disability* compiled by Michael Mandelstam, published by the Disabled Living Foundation.

ℹ *Directory of Aids for Disabled People* by Ann Darnborough and Derek Kinrade, published by Woodhead Faulkner.

ℹ *A Guide to Grants for Individuals in Need*, published by the Directory of Social Change.

Accommodation

Independent living

Independent living – that is, living in their own home – is likely to be the preferred option of most people with arthritis. Community care aims to facilitate this. Mobility problems are rarely insurmountable – a little ingenuity can go a long way – and social services are not the only body who may be able to help, as outlined in Chapter 4.

What, then, are the likely problems with independent living? Everyday tasks may be difficult: some may need to be done by someone else. The risk of accidents is real enough – probably far greater than the risk of crime. Loneliness can be overcome if family and friends live nearby and can visit regularly. By contrast, the advantages of not having to move and remaining independent in familiar surroundings are obvious.

Practical help in the home is discussed in Chapter 4; here we look at how the home can be adapted to make it more suitable. If major adaptations are being considered, information and advice on design issues and a database of architects, surveyors and similar professionals with experience of designing for disabled people are available from the Centre for Accessible Environments (address on p 151).

Grants for alterations are available from the local authority, but they depend on the claimant's income and savings. Most grants are *discretionary*, meaning that it is up to the local authority to decide whether to give them. A few grants for necessary adaptations for disabled people are *mandatory*, meaning that the local authority must give the grant to anyone who qualifies.

Grants made under the Home Energy Efficiency scheme are available to anyone aged over 60, to help with home insulation. People receiving certain state benefits will get the maximum grant (£315 in 1999); others get 25 per cent of the maximum.

Renovation grants are used to pay for essential repairs or to provide essential services such as an indoor toilet or a bath or shower with hot and cold water.

Home repair assistance grants are available for smaller repairs and alterations (these grants are not available in Scotland). They are also given for alterations to enable a person aged 60 or over to move into a carer's home; for example, installing a downstairs toilet. If the work costs more than the amount of the grant (in 1999: £2,000 per individual application or £4,000 over three years), you will have to make up the difference yourself.

Disabled facilities grants, as their name suggests, are given to provide facilities for a disabled person. They are mandatory if they are for specified purposes, including improved access to and in the home, improving or adapting heating or safety and providing facilities for independent living. The local authority usually requires an assessment by an occupational therapist confirming that the adaptations are necessary.

Note *Never* start the work before getting the local authority's approval to go ahead, or you will not be entitled to a grant.

Brenda has rheumatoid arthritis and is cared for by her husband Tom.

Brenda

'We've had a lot of adaptations made to our house. The local authority have helped with some but not all and it's not been cheap. The alterations to the bathroom cost £3,400, and the firm didn't even redecorate.

'You need to be very careful. I saw one advert in a paper that said the company was recommended by Arthritis Care. I phoned the charity and they said it wasn't.'

Don't forget how much the local authority can help.

Tom

'We live in Lambeth, which must be one of the most criticised boroughs in the country but, once Brenda was registered disabled, we only had to wait four weeks before they painted a parking bay outside our house. They also fitted rails outside – we live on quite a steep hill – and smaller ones throughout the house. They also put an extra banister on the stairs. I knew all this was available because I used to do this sort of work myself when I worked at the local hospital.'

Brenda again

'We were lucky. Tom met an occupational therapist at an Arthritis Care meeting and she came round and had a look for us. One of the problems with rheumatologists is that they don't always tell the occupational therapist about you or you about them. Make sure you ask about them.'

Reducing accidents

We all know the home can be a dangerous place but a little thought can make it much safer.

- Falls are usually caused by tripping, so grab rails are really useful.
- Keep the floors in living areas free from clutter.
- Trailing flexes can be tacked to the wall, or more sockets installed.
- Go for simple floor-coverings. Fitted carpets are safer than slippery floors
- If there are mats, make sure they have non-slip strips fitted.
- Worn stair carpet is particularly dangerous.
- Reducing the need for stretching and reaching will also reduce the likelihood of accidents, so think about locations and accessibility of shelves and cupboards.
- The impact of falls can be reduced by cushioning sharp edges and avoiding low level glass unless it is safety glass.
- Non-safety glass can be coated with a shatterproof film to make it safer.
- Plenty of lights with easy-to-use rocker or touch-sensitive switches will help.
- Make sure that handles are easy to use and move readily. Long handles that are easier to turn are available for doors and taps.

Most accidents happen in the kitchen and bathroom. An accident in the kitchen is usually the result of knocking against something or trying to lift something too heavy; in the bathroom, from trying to manoeuvre in a small room with a slippery floor. To prevent accidents, think about how these rooms will be used. Work step by step through each process. Most problems can be solved. For example, instead of lifting a heavy pan of vegetables from the cooker to the sink, use a wire mesh basket of the type often used for chips to lift the vegetables out of the water. Make sure that all gas and electric appliances are checked regularly, and fit smoke alarms. Think about other gadgets that could reduce the risk of accidents – pill reminders, alarms, carbon monoxide detectors and so on.

For more *i*nformation

ℹ️ For more information on independent living, contact the National Centre for Independent Living (address on p 156), which can direct you to your local Centre.

ℹ️ Age Concern Factsheet 13 *Older home owners: financial help with repairs and adaptations.*

ℹ️ Age Concern Factsheet 42 *Disability equipment and how to get it.*

ℹ️ For more advice on preventing accidents, contact the Royal Society for the Prevention of Accidents (RoSPA) (address on p 158).

ℹ️ *Take Care With Arthritis* is a useful leaflet produced by Arthritis Care.

Sheltered accommodation

This type of accommodation can be an option that gives the best of both worlds, providing much of the independence of living in one's own home but with a warden nearby. The properties are usually purpose-built blocks of flats or bungalows designed with disability in mind. Sheltered housing is offered by local authorities, commercial companies and also by housing associations. Some properties are available to rent, others to buy; there may be other options, such as shared ownership, leasehold and so on.

But there are some aspects to think carefully about. If the person with arthritis is considering buying, what exactly are they getting for their money? Some of these properties may not be particularly good value compared with others in the area, and whilst an older buyer will be thinking about present benefits rather than future investment, there is no point in paying over the odds. Whether renting or buying, it is important to know exactly what degree of shelter is being offered. Some include a restaurant and other facilities, whereas others offer little more than an alarm system. Whatever the case, how does the alarm work and when is the warden on site?

Check out the hidden costs such as maintenance charges very carefully. There may be a number of these, and they may rise sharply.

131

The local environment is also important, as it is whenever we move home. What facilities are nearby – shops, banks, post office, pharmacist/chemist shop, library, doctor's surgery, clubs, pubs, day centres, cinemas and so on? What transport is available? Is the area too hilly?

There are two codes of practice to look out for: the National House Building Council (NHBC) Sheltered Housing Code of Practice, which covers the building of properties; and the Association of Retirement Housing Managers Code of Practice, which covers the way in which they are managed. Under the NHBC code, purchasers should be given an information pack outlining exactly what, in terms of property and services, is being provided and by whom.

The local authority's housing department should be able to give information about sheltered accommodation in their area. Age Concern and the Elderly Accommodation Counsel (address on p 154) can also provide advice. Sheltered accommodation with extra arthritis care is provided by the Abbeyfield Society, usually in larger houses converted into a number of bed-sitters.

Moving in with you

Moving someone with care needs into your home may seem like the obvious option but it is a big step for both of you. The privacy and independence of both parties is compromised and your relationship is complicated. It may be a very thorny issue when the person needing care is a relative. Some people have strong views about the role of family members, particularly that of women, and their obligations in caring for others in the family. You may hold some of these. So may the relative who needs care. Being open and talking it through is really the only way to address these issues.

Feeling that you don't want your relative to move in with you is nothing to be ashamed of. You get only one life and you have a right to yours, as have the other people who already live with you. Nobody should enter into this sort of arrangement just because they can't say 'No'. If the relationship is not strong enough for one of you to say 'I don't want to live with you', it doesn't bode well for living together.

In any event, a trial period is a good idea – call it a holiday. If you do go down this route, your home may need some adaptations: see the section on adaptations (including grants for these) on page 121.

Another possibility, if finances permit, is to build an annexe to your home for the person with arthritis to move into. This can provide the ideal compromise, giving you both independence while maintaining close contact.

Residential care

People often regard 'going into a home' as a last resort, and may be sceptical about the quality and value of the care provided. Nevertheless, there are homes that provide good care, and one of those might be the best option. Independence is lost but, in a good home, probably not to the degree that might be feared. Carers are strangers – which some people regard as an advantage – and they ought to be professionals.

If this is the option the person with arthritis prefers, the best thing you can do as a carer is to ensure that the home and its facilities are thoroughly checked out. There are care homes run by the private sector, by voluntary organisations and by the local authority. Many homes in the voluntary sector are for particular groups of people – war veterans, for example; one of these may be appropriate.

The best way to find a home is probably by word of mouth but social workers, health professionals and local voluntary organisations can also help. The registration officer for residential care homes at the local authority social services department will have a list of local homes. They might also be able to help by arranging visits to a home – particularly if they are suggesting a care home following a social services assessment – and showing you the latest local authority inspection report on how the home is run. The health authority's registration officer for nursing homes will have a list of nursing homes.

It is vital to visit the homes being considered. Some will prefer you to make an appointment but others will suggest that you call in any time. It may be possible for the person with arthritis to arrange to stay for a short 'holiday', to get a better feel of the home before making a final decision.

Issues to consider

- The 'ethos' of the home – do they encourage residents to make their own decisions? Can they, for example, eat what they want? Is there a residents' committee?
- Privacy – private phones? Single or shared rooms? What about personal possessions?
- Flexibility – how fixed are visiting times, bed times, meal times and so on?
- Facilities – for example, are there outings and recreational opportunities, communal living rooms, books, newspapers, mobile library?
- Cost – the contract between the home and the resident should state clearly the fees and what extras might apply.
- Environment – the considerations of access to local shops and transport and so on, discussed under sheltered accommodation (p 131), apply here too.

Paying for (permanent) residential care

Residential homes can be paid for in three ways:

- By the local authority if a care home is suggested following a social services assessment. In this case the resident would pay a fee based on national rules, which may be less than the commercial cost of the care. These rules, explained in detail below, take account of:
  - income, including most benefits and pensions;
  - capital, including savings, investments and the value of any property (someone with capital over £16,000 is expected to pay the full cost);

The individual should be able to opt for a different home – called their 'preferred accommodation' – but might have to make up the difference if the home is more expensive than the local authority would normally pay.

■ By the health authority if the person meets the eligibility criteria. In this case the NHS meets costs but the resident remains a hospital patient with all the limits on their pension and benefit entitlement that this involves. Every health authority should have a written statement on their 'Policy and Eligibility Criteria for Continuing Health Care', which explains who needs continuing in-patient care and how decisions about it will be taken.

■ Privately.

Paying for local-authority-funded residential care

Generally, most of the resident's income – including most Social Security benefits such as Incapacity Benefit, Income Support, the state pension and any company or personal pension – goes towards the cost of care. Half of a private pension (ie an occupational pension, a personal pension or a retirement annuity) will be ignored, provided that it is going to a spouse. A spouse at home can be asked to make a contribution, although local authorities can use their discretion to ensure that the husband or wife remaining at home has reasonable income to pay for living expenses if the resident has the majority of the couple's income.

When the local authority is funding residential care, Attendance Allowance will cease to be paid after four weeks (or sooner following a stay in hospital). If the local authority stops funding residential care, Attendance Allowance will be restored.

Social services' calculations will ensure that a resident retains a sum of money each week, known as the 'personal allowance', to cover personal expenses. The resident will also have any other income or capital that is not counted under the rules mentioned above. The personal allowance can be increased in certain circumstances – for example, to prepare someone for more

135

independent living by encouraging them to manage their own finances or to take account of any family commitments.

The local authority should be able to advise whether a resident is likely to qualify for Income Support. The main criteria are: savings of less than £16,000 for a permanent resident or less than £8,000 for someone in residential care only temporarily. Claims for Income Support are made to the local Benefits Agency office.

For the purpose of calculating fees, capital is ignored up to a certain level (£10,000 in 1999) but a rate of income is assumed on all savings above this amount. This capital includes the value of any home the resident owns unless it is still occupied:

- by their husband or wife or a partner who lived with them as if married;
- by a relative who is 60 or over, or under 60 but incapacitated;
- by a relative who is under 16 and whom the resident is legally liable to support.

If the house has other occupants, social services have the discretion to exclude the home's value.

If the home's value is taken into account, it may be necessary to sell it in order to realise the capital but that is up to the individual. There may be another way to meet the fees. The local authority may place a 'legal charge' on a property, enabling it to recoup anything it is owed in the event of its sale sometime in the future.

Some people may try to give away property or other capital before an assessment is made. The moral issues of this aside, social services can still take that property or capital into account if they consider that it was given away to avoid paying the proper contribution.

Paying for residential care privately

Even someone who can arrange and pay for a care home themselves is advised not to move into one until they have asked social services for an assessment. A residential home may not be the best option. Social services may be able suggest ways that would allow continued independent living. They will also be happy to give provide information about homes, including their reports on them, to people arranging their own care.

Anyone making their own arrangements should also think about what might happen as their money runs out. It may be possible to stay in the home chosen but, if social services consider that it is not suitable or it costs too much, they may arrange a place elsewhere. If it is likely that capital will fall below £16,000, it is sensible to talk to the social services department before moving into a home.

If property is being sold to pay for a move into care, both Income Support and Attendance Allowance may be claimed. It should be possible to find a private or voluntary care home that will agree to make special arrangements until a resident's own home is sold. Once the property is sold, Income Support will stop if the person's capital is now over £16,000.

It is possible to take out insurance against needing to move into residential care in the future. If you or the person with arthritis are considering this, it is important to seek independent advice and to check exactly what is covered by the policy.

The Royal Commission on Long-term Care

The Royal Commission on Long-term Care, which reported in the spring of 1999, suggested changes in the funding for long-term care. It said that housing and living costs should be means-tested and that personal and health care should be free. At the time of writing, the Government was encouraging debate on the Commission's report.

For more *i*nformation

ⓘ Age Concern Factsheet 2 *Retirement housing for sale.*

ⓘ Age Concern Factsheet 8 *Moving into rented housing.*

ⓘ Age Concern Factsheet 10 *Local authority charging procedures for residential and nursing home care.*

- ℹ️ Age Concern Factsheet 29 *Finding residential and nursing home accommodation.*

- ℹ️ Age Concern Factsheet 38 *Treatment of the former home as capital for people in residential and nursing homes.*

- ℹ️ Age Concern Factsheet 39 *Paying for care in a residential or nursing home if you have a partner.*

- ℹ️ Age Concern Factsheet 40 *Transfer of assets and paying for care in a residential or nursing home.*

Getting about

By car

Many people with arthritis can drive. Often, all that is needed are a few features that are now standard on many cars – power steering and automatic transmission, for example. There is also an abundance of adaptations and aids available, which means that even the most specialist needs can be met.

When buying or leasing a car, it is vital to try it out thoroughly, having made sure that it meets all needs. Consider, for example, whether the car should have two or four doors: in a two-door car, the seat can be slid further back and the door is usually bigger and opens wider; but this will make the door heavier and perhaps more difficult to shut. Look out also for the door sills: high sills can make it harder to get in and out of the car. And how easy will it be to load and unload a wheelchair? A very good way to find out what one's needs are is to get an assessment from an approved mobility centre. For more information about cars and assessments, contact the Mobility Advice and Vehicle Information Service (MAVIS) at Crowthorne or the Banstead Mobility Centre.

People receiving the higher rate of the mobility component of the Disability Living Allowance (see pp 110–111) can generally use it to buy or lease a car from Motability, the government initiative to get disabled people mobile.

Concessions that may be available to disabled motorists include:

- exemption from road tax if the vehicle is used exclusively by or for a disabled person (contact the DLA Unit of the Department of Social Security (address on p 160, under 'Vehicle Excise Duty') for information);
- the use of disabled parking bays;
- the Orange Badge scheme (Blue Badge from 2000) which, with a few exceptions, allows parking in otherwise restricted areas such as on yellow lines; applications are made to the local authority social services department, which can supply an explanatory leaflet *The Orange Badge Scheme.*

By public transport

With privatisation and deregulation, it is hard to make generalisations about the quality of public transport for disabled people. The Government has issued guidelines for new buses, coaches, taxis and trains to be more accessible for disabled passengers. However, it will be many years before all vehicles comply.

Rail operators say most of the trains in use today have fold-up seats to allow a space for wheelchair-users. In first class, wheelchairs can be moved up and down the carriages, but not in standard class or in the buffet area. Operators say that most Intercity services are fitted with automatic doors inside to allow easy movement in the train, and there is an assistance button by the wheelchair space which will call the senior conductor.

Railtrack (which controls most stations) say that many stations have ramps that allow wheelchairs to be wheeled onto trains. Their advice is 'Just ask any member of staff for assistance at stations.' Most companies will meet you at stations and provide assistance if you telephone in advance (preferably giving 48 hours' notice), but assistance will normally be provided even if no warning is given. Many major stations have lifts to each platform and many other smaller stations have ramps to platforms. Staff can radio ahead to ensure that there is somebody waiting to meet you with another ramp at the destination station. Unfortunately, there is no facility

139

for coping with people's specific needs at unstaffed stations; the only choice is usually to travel from and to staffed stations.

Disabled-accessible toilets are provided at many stations. Trains are being refurbished to provide disabled-accessible toilets. At the moment, though, there is no way of knowing whether there will be any on a particular train.

Local rail operators should produce leaflets about their facilities for disabled people, including the Disabled Persons Railcard. RADAR produce *A Guide to British Rail for Disabled People*, which gives access details about over 500 stations. For further information, telephone National Rail Enquiries on 0345 48 49 50.

Contact the local bus company for details of accessible buses. Some operators use vehicles that meet some or all of the access standards of the Disabled Persons Transport Advisory Committee, such as low steps, handrails and bells that are easy to push. Some cities have Mobility Buses, which are accessible to people in wheelchairs. Dial-a-Ride schemes, which enable disabled people to book lifts in a minibus or similar vehicle, are available in many areas. The local disability advice organisation should be able to provide more information.

Airlines are also becoming more aware of the needs of disabled people. The key point here, as with all public transport, is to be very specific in advance about what is needed and when. For example, what arrangements need to be made for a wheelchair? Your travel agent should be able to tell you what facilities are available. It is probably worth double-checking with the airline and/or the airport nearer the departure time to make sure that the relevant people have been informed (or have not forgotten) about any requirements.

As with other forms of transport, facilities for people with disabilities when travelling by ship can vary widely, both at terminals and on board. Check with the travel agent and/or the shipping company to find out what facilities are available and to let them know of any requirements for you or the person you are caring for.

It is irritating that few transport operators seem able to offer the sort of blanket access that would enable disabled people to use their facilities on the same basis as non-disabled people. However, with advance warning their 'customer care' strategies come into play and most will try to be helpful.

Although disabled people should not be discriminated against in transport services, the Disability Discrimination Act excludes the right to accessible transport. Nevertheless, be clear with transport operators about what is required. They, like you, know that TV's *Watchdog* programme and the rest of the consumer media and consumer organisations are only a phone call away.

Schemes to help with transport

- Dial-a-Ride and Community Transport schemes provide a door-to-door service for shopping or similar outings for people who cannot use public transport (addresses on pp 152 and 151).
- Hospital Car schemes are usually run by the ambulance service and arranged through the GP surgery. They are only for someone who has a medical condition and cannot get to the hospital independently; one companion is usually allowed.
- Shopmobility schemes are available in many town centres. They will lend a wheelchair/scooter to anyone with a mobility problem. The user can often park free or be met at the bus station or taxi rank by prior arrangement.
- Taxicard (or similar name) is a service that provides subsidised taxi fares; it is run by some larger local authorities for disabled people who cannot use public transport. One passenger may accompany the cardholder. The local council office should have information about this.
- Tripscope (address on p 159) specialise in giving information and advice on travel and transport for older and disabled people. They are not a travel or booking agency but can help you plan a journey so that it will be as easy as possible.

In shops

Shops vary widely in accessibility. Although many can be entered relatively easily, even with a wheelchair, the aisles may be narrow and difficult to manoeuvre in. Some supermarkets now have trolleys that can be used with a wheelchair but there remains the difficulty of getting items out of reach if the person with arthritis is unaccompanied.

Larger shops often have chairs for their customers but it may be worth asking smaller shops without any already set out to make a chair available.

For more *information*

i Age Concern Factsheet 26 *Travel information for older people.*

i *Getting There: A guide to long distance travel for disabled people,* published by RADAR.

i For information about local schemes to help with transport, contact the local council.

Taking a break

Taking a break – or respite care – is often cited by carers as the single most important thing in making their job possible. Tony has been married for 56 years to Sheila and now cares for her. He thinks a little time apart is invaluable.

Tony

'We have a Crossroads carer once a week and a daily paid carer, which takes a lot of the weight off my shoulders. It gives us both our own time. I like to paint, read or do crosswords. It's imperative to have a break, even from the person you love most in the world.'

Tom and teenager Jenny agree.

Tom

'The toughest thing about caring is not getting a break. I don't mind taking care of everything on a day-to-day basis – that keeps me busy – but it's the fact that it never stops. As you get older you have less energy and get tired. We haven't had a holiday since I retired. I think I'm pretty resourceful and our generation are good at making do but even so ...'

Jenny

'I'm involved with the Edinburgh Young Carers group so I can chat and go out with other people in the same position. That helps a lot. But a befriender to take my mum out too would really make a difference.'

Everybody needs some time off occasionally – and if you're a carer you need it more than most. But the Carers National Association reckon that over half of those who spend more than 20 hours a week caring haven't had even a couple of days off since they started caring. And some carers even feel guilty for wanting a break.

If you feel like this, let your guilt go and examine the situation objectively. Without a break, any human being will become tired. If you are tired, you can make mistakes or become ill – two things that are no good at all for you or the person you are caring for. If that doesn't convince you, what about the benefits to the other person? They could do with a break from you too. A change of scene, some time with other people, and you'll both feel better afterwards.

The options for breaks include care at home, day care away from home, residential breaks and holidays.

Care at home

Under the Carers Act you have a right to have your needs assessed, and one of these could well be the need for a break. Social services may offer home help, meals-on-wheels or a sitter or care attendant. If necessary, point out to them the advantages to their budget of supporting you as a carer now, rather than meeting the full care costs of the person you care for in the future because you cannot cope. GPs may be able to arrange some care at home, such as visits from the district nurse to help with nursing care.

If another member of your family or a friend cannot stand in for you, explore local sitting services. Many social services, health authorities and voluntary organisations can provide sitters, offering helpers for a few hours a week. They can just sit with the person or they may provide help with getting up or preparing meals. Most are experienced although untrained. There may be a charge. For more care, consider a local authority care attendant. Again, there may be a charge.

Crossroads Care has the largest network of voluntary schemes – around 230 in the UK – and the Leonard Cheshire Foundation also has a Care At Home service. The Community Service Volunteers can also match volunteers with organisations or people needing help.

Day care away from home

This can be a regular daily or weekly break or a week every few months. It may be provided by voluntary organisations, by the health or local authority, by a government scheme or by the local education authority. There might be a charge. Day care can be at a day centre or a lunch and social club, or at a day hospital if specialist medical treatment or care is needed. There are also education, training and work centres. Transport may be provided, for which there may be a charge.

Residential breaks

To get a good break for a few days, there is the possibility of temporary residential care for the person for whom you care. It will give you both a change, and give you the house to yourself for a while if you live together.

It may involve a short stay in a hospital, a hospice or a residential or nursing home. Respite stays in an NHS hospital or a hospice run by a charity are usually free. If the local authority arranges a stay in a residential or nursing home, there will usually be a flat-rate nightly fee. For a stay over eight weeks, there will normally be a means test. There are a few schemes enabling the person you care for to stay with another family. These are mainly for children but there are some for adults. Ask social services about family-based respite care whereby people go and stay with another carefully selected and trained family.

Holidays

You can go on holiday either together or separately. There is a little financial help available, although eligibility criteria can be strict. There are home exchange schemes and some holiday companies that specialise in singles or in special needs. These are listed in the Carers National Association leaflet *Taking a Break*.

Organising a break can be expensive, which is another good reason to make sure you are claiming all the benefits you are both entitled to. Charities may be able to help too. Consult the book *A Guide to Grants for Individuals in Need* in your local library.

RADAR publish several holiday guides, giving information on places to stay in the UK (including information on the availability of ground-floor bedrooms, lifts, size of entrance doors), holidays in the rest of Europe, access to air travel, ferries, rail and coach travel and insurance. The Holiday Care Service (address on p 155) is a charity that provides specialist travel and holiday information for disabled people and their carers. They publish a variety of information sheets on topics such as how to find voluntary or paid helpers/carers for holidays and travel, and finding help towards the cost of a holiday. They also have a reservations service for accessible hotels in the UK. Tripscope provide a telephone information service, giving advice on most aspects of travel and transport for older and disabled people. It includes journey planning, where to hire a wheelchair on holiday, the location of the local Dial-a-Ride and where to find an escort to help someone across a major city.

For further *i*nformation

ℹ️ For more on respite care, contact Crossroads Care or the Leonard Cheshire Foundation, which run the UK 'Care At Home' service. The Community Service Volunteers can also provide volunteers. (See the 'Useful addresses' section for details of these organisations.)

ℹ️ *Residential and Nursing Home Care*, a booklet produced by Carers National Association.

ℹ️ RADAR (address on p 158) publish several holiday guides and holiday fact packs:

Accessible Holidays in the British Isles 1999: A guide for disabled people;

Access to Air Travel: A guide for first time disabled travellers;

European Holidays and Travel Abroad 1998;

Getting There: A guide to long distance travel for disabled people;

Fact pack 1: *General information*;

Fact pack 2: *Transport and equipment*;

Fact pack 3: *Holiday alternatives*.

ℹ️ Contact Tripscope for advice about travel and transport (address on p 159).

7 Five things for every carer

I hope this book hasn't put you off becoming a carer but, rather, has helped you appreciate exactly what is being taken on and suggested ways to help you cope with the challenges. Probably the five most useful things a carer can do are summarised here.

- Get a carer's assessment from the local social services department. They can assess the type of support you need, such as meals-on-wheels, respite care and practical help in the home. This assessment is your right under the Carers Act.
- Find out about – and use – respite care.
- Make sure that your doctor, social services, pharmacist and employer know your situation.
- Talk about how you feel with someone in the family who understands the situation or with a close friend, GP or counsellor. Try the Arthritis Care Freephone Helpline 0808 800 4050 (Monday–Friday 12–4) or the Carers National Association CarersLine 0345 573 369 (Monday–Friday 10–12; 2–4) – calls at local rates.
- Check out what the Carers National Association can offer. It has 120 branches in the UK. For your nearest group, call 020 7490 8818. You should certainly make sure you join some sort of an organisation or group where you can meet other carers, while encouraging the person you are caring for to join a group such as Arthritis Care where they can meet other people with arthritis.

Useful addresses

Abbeyfield Society
53 Victoria Street
St Albans
Herts AL1 3UW
Tel: 01727 857536

Housing association specialising in bedsitters for older people in shared houses, with meals provided.

Air Transport Users Council
CAA House
45–59 Kingsway
London WC2B 6TE
Tel: 020 7240 6061

Publish a booklet Flight Plan, *which has a section for disabled passengers.*

Arthritis Care
18 Stephenson Way
London NW1 2HD
Tel: 020 7916 1500
Freephone helpline 0808 800 4050 (Monday–Friday 12–4pm)

Provide information, counselling, training, fun and social contact. The first port of call for anyone with arthritis. There are many smaller organisations for particular types of arthritis. Arthritis Care's helpline can provide details.

Arthritis Research Campaign
Copeman House
St Mary's Court
St Mary's Gate
Chesterfield S41 7TD
Tel: 01246 558033
Website: http://www.arc.org.uk/
The leading arthritis research organisation in the UK, funding much research and also producing useful information for patients.

Association of Reflexologists
27 Old Gloucester Street
London WC1N 3XX
Tel: 0870 567 3320
The largest independent organisation of reflexologists.

Association of Traditional Chinese Medicine
78 Haverstock Hill
London NW3 2BE
Tel: 020 7284 2898

Many Chinese-trained practitioners of herbal medicine are members.

Banstead Mobility Centre
Damson Way
Fountains Drive
Carshalton
Surrey SM5 4NR
Tel: 020 8770 1151
For driving assessment and advice.

Benefits Enquiry Line
Tel: 0800 88 22 00
Website: http://www/dss/gov/uk/ba
State benefits information line for sick or disabled people and their carers.

British Acupuncture Council
63 Jeddo Road
London W12 9HQ
Tel: 020 8735 0400
Fax: 020 8735 0404
Regulatory body of acupuncturists.

British Association for Counselling
1 Regent Place
Rugby
Warwickshire CV21 2PJ
Tel: 01788 578328 (Helpline)
Publish a directory of counsellors in the UK. Send an sae for information.

British Chiropractic Association
Blagrave House
17 Blagrave Street
Reading RG1 1QB
Freephone: 0800 212 618
Regulatory body of chiropractors.

British Homoeopathic Association
27a Devonshire Street
London W1N 1RJ
Tel: 020 7935 2163
One of two regulatory bodies of homoeopaths; members are also trained doctors. Send sae (60p) for information.

Carers National Association
20–25 Glasshouse Yard
London EC1A 4JS
Tel: 020 7490 8818
CarersLine 0345 573 369 (Monday–Friday 10am–12 noon; 2–4pm; calls at local rates)
Provide a wide range of information and support to all carers.

Centre for Accessible Environments
Nutmeg House
60 Gainsford Street
London SE1 2NY
Tel: 020 7357 8182

Give advice on accessible design for buildings.

Chartered Society of Physiotherapy
14 Bedford Row
London WC1R 4ED
Tel: 020 7242 1941

For chartered physiotherapists in your area.

College of Health National Waiting Lists Helpline
Tel: 020 8983 1133

Can sometimes find a shorter waiting list for hospital treatment.

Community Service Volunteers
237 Pentonville Road
London N1 9NJ
Tel: 020 7278 6601

Can provide voluntary care assistants.

Community Transport Association
Highbank
Halton Street
Hyde
Cheshire SK14 2NY
Tel: 0161 351 1475
Advice: 0161 367 8780

Services to benefit providers of transport for people with mobility problems.

Crossroads Care
(Association of Crossroads Care Attendants Schemes Ltd)
10 Regent Place
Rugby
Warwickshire CV21 2PN
Tel: England: 01788 573653
    Wales: 01222 222282
    Scotland: 0141 226 3793
    Northern Ireland: 028 9181 4455

For a care attendant to come into your home and look after your relative.

Department of Health
PO Box 410
Wetherby LS23 7LN

For a free copy of the introductory Guide to Receiving Direct Payments.

Dial-a-Ride (DART)
Unit 11
Spectrum House
32–34 Gordon House Road
London NW5 1LP
Tel: 020 7482 2325

Campaign for accessible transport for older and disabled people. Offer information about local Dial-a-Ride and Taxicard schemes.

Disability Alliance
Universal House
88–94 Wentworth Street
London E1 7SA
Tel: 020 7247 8776
Helpline: 020 7247 8763 (Monday and Wednesday 2–4pm)

Information on welfare benefits.

Disability Information and Advice Lines (DIAL)
DIAL UK
Park Lodge
St Catherine's Hospital
Tickhill Road
Balby
Doncaster DN4 8QN
Tel: 01302 310 123

For your nearest local group, giving information and advice about disability.

Disability Sport England
13–27 Brunswick Place
London N1 6DX
Tel: 020 7490 4919

National events agency that encourages sport from local to national level.

Disabled Living Centres Council
Redbank House
4 St Chad's Street
Manchester M8 8QA
Tel: 0161 834 1044

For a Centre near you, where you can see aids and equipment.

Disabled Living Foundation
380–384 Harrow Road
London W9 2HU
Tel: 020 7289 6111
Helpline: 0870 603 9177
Website: http://www.dlf.org.uk/

Information and advice about aids to help people cope with a disability.

Disabled Persons Railcard Office
PO Box 1YT
Newcastle-upon-Tyne NE99 1YT
Helpline: 0191 269 0303

For a railcard offering concessionary fares. An application form and booklet Rail Travel for Disabled Passengers *can be found at most staffed stations or from the address above.*

Disablement Income Group
PO Box 5743
Finchingfield
Essex CM7 4PW
Tel: 01371 811621

Advice and research aiming to improve the income of disabled people.

Elderly Accommodation Counsel
3rd Floor
89 Albert Embankment
London SE1 7TP
Tel: 020 7820 1343
Helpline: 020 7820 3970

Computerised information about all forms of accommodation for older people (including nursing homes and hospices) and advice on top-up funding.

English Heritage
23 Savile Row
London W1X 1AB
Tel: 020 7973 3434

For a guide for people with disabilities.

Financial Services Authority/Public Investment Authority
25 The North Colonnade
Canary Wharf
London E14 5HS
Tel: 020 7676 1000

Regulates the investment industry.

General Chiropractic Council
344–354 Gray's Inn Road
London WC1X 8BT
Tel: 020 7713 5155

The statutory body regulating practitioners of chiropractic.

General Osteopathic Council
Osteopathic House
176 Tower Bridge Road
London SE1 3LU
Tel: 020 7357 6655
Regulatory body of osteopaths.

Holiday Care Service
2nd floor, Imperial Buildings
Victoria Road
Horley
Surrey RH6 7PZ
Tel: 01293 774535
Free information and advice about holidays for disabled people and their carers.

Independent Living (1993) Fund
PO Box 183
Nottingham NG8 3RD
Tel: 0115 942 8191/2
May fund very severely disabled people to buy in extra care.

Institute for Complementary Medicine
PO Box 194
London SE16 1QZ
Tel: 020 7237 5165 (weekdays 10am–2pm)
Information and advice about complementary therapy. (Please send self-addressed envelope and two 2nd class stamps.)

Leonard Cheshire Foundation
30 Millbank
London SW1P 4QD
Tel: 020 7802 8200
Residential homes and home care attendants for disabled people.

MAVIS (Mobility Advice and Vehicle Information Service)
O Wing
Macadam Avenue
Old Wokingham Road
Crowthorne
Berks RG45 6XD
Tel: 01344 661000
Driving assessments and advice.

Motability
Goodman House
Station Approach
Harlow
Essex CM20 2ET
Tel: 01279 635 999
Helpline: 01279 635 666
Advice and help about cars, scooters and wheelchairs for disabled people.

Naidex
Touchstone Exhibitions and Conferences
Haleon House
4 Red Lion Street
Richmond
Surrey TW9 1RW
Tel: 020 8332 0044
Runs exhibitions at which manufacturers of aids and equipment can show their wares.

National Centre for Independent Living
250 Kennington Lane
London SE11 5RD
Tel: 020 7587 1663

Provides advice on independent living and direct payments, and details of your local Centre for Independent Living.

National Health Service information service
0800 66 55 44
First point of contact to find out about NHS services.

National Institute of Medical Herbalists
56 Longbrook Street
Exeter
Devon EX4 6AH
Tel: 01392 426022
Regulatory body of practitioners of Western herbal medicine.

National Rail Enquiries
Tel: 0345 48 49 50
For information about facilities for disabled people.

National Trust Disability Office
36 Queen Anne's Gate
London SW1H 9AS
Tel: 020 7447 6742/3
For the booklet on National Trust properties, Information for Visitors with Disabilities.

Occupational Pensions Regulatory Authority
Invicta House
Trafalgar Place
Brighton
East Sussex BN1 4DW
Tel: 01273 627600
The statutory regulator for the operation of occupational pension schemes in the UK.

Princess Royal Trust for Carers
142 Minories
London EC3N 1LB
Tel: 020 7480 7788
Fax: 020 7481 4729
Aims to make it easier for carers to cope by providing information, support and practical help. Your phone book may list a local branch.

Psoriatic Arthropathy Alliance
PO Box 111
St Albans
Herts AL2 3JQ
Tel: 01923 682606
Fax: 01923 672837
Helps people with psoriatic arthritis, and raises awareness of the condition.

RADAR (Royal Association for Disability and Rehabilitation)
12 City Forum
250 City Road
London EC1V 8AF
Tel: 020 7250 3222
Textphone: 020 7250 4119
Information and publications about aids and mobility, holidays and leisure.

> *Northern Ireland:*
> **Disability Action**
> 2 Annadale Avenue
> Belfast BT7 3JH
> Tel: 028 9049 1011
>
> *Scotland:*
> **Disability Scotland**
> Princes House
> 5 Shandwick Place
> Edinburgh EH2 4RG
> Tel: 0131 229 8632
>
> *Wales:*
> **Disability Wales**
> Llys Ifor, Crescent Road
> Caerphilly CF83 1XL
> Tel: 029 2088 7325

REMAP GB
National Co-ordinator
Hazeldene
Ightham
Sevenoaks
Kent TN15 9AD
Tel: 01732 883818
For customised aids and gadgets.

RoSPA (Royal Society for the Prevention of Accidents)
Edgbaston Park
353 Bristol Road
Birmingham B5 7ST
Tel: 0121 248 2000
Advice and publications on preventing accidents.

Society of Homoeopaths
2 Artizan Road
Northampton NN1 4HU
Tel: 01604 621400

One of two regulatory bodies of homoeopaths.

Sport England (formerly **Sports Council**)
16 Upper Woburn Place
London WC1H 0QP
Tel: 020 7273 1500

For addresses of regional sports councils.

Thrive (formerly **Horticultural Therapy**)
Geoffrey Udall Centre
Trunkwell Park
Beech Hill
Reading RG7 2AT
Tel: 0118 988 5688

Advice, information and training on gardening for people with disabilities or special needs.

Tripscope (London)
The Courtyard
Evelyn Road
London W4 5JL
Tel/Textphone: 08457 585641

A travel and transport information service for older and disabled people.

UK Home Care Association (UKHCA)
42b Banstead Road
Carshalton Beeches
Surrey SM5 3NW
Tel: 020 8288 1551

For information about organisations providing home care in your area.

Vehicle Excise Duty (road tax)
DLA Unit
Warbreck House
Warbreck Hill Road
Blackpool FY2 0YE
Tel: 01345 123456

Information about exemption from road tax for vehicles used exclusively by or for disabled people.

West of England Centre for Independent Living
Leinster Avenue
Knowle
Bristol BS4 1AR
Tel: 0117 983 9839

Advice and a guide for users of the direct payments scheme, Personal Assistants Employer's Handbook.

About Age Concern

Caring for someone with arthritis is one of a wide range of publications produced by Age Concern England, the National Council on Ageing. Age Concern cares about all older people and believes that later life should be fulfilling and enjoyable. For too many this is impossible. As the leading charitable movement in the UK concerned with ageing and older people, Age Concern finds effective ways to change that situation.

Where possible, we enable older people to solve problems themselves, providing as much or as little support as they need. Our network of 1,400 local groups, supported by 250,000 volunteers, provides community-based services such as lunch clubs, day centres and home visiting.

Nationally, we take a lead role in campaigning, parliamentary work, policy analysis, research, specialist information and advice provision, and publishing. Innovative programmes promote healthier lifestyles and provide older people with opportunities to give the experience of a lifetime back to their communities.

Age Concern is dependent on donations, covenants and legacies.

Age Concern England
1268 London Road
London SW16 4ER
Tel: 020 8765 7211
Fax: 020 8765 7211

Age Concern Scotland
113 Rose Street
Edinburgh EH2 3DT
Tel: 0131 220 3345
Fax: 0131 220 2779

Age Concern Cymru
4th Floor
1 Cathedral Road
Cardiff CF1 9SD
Tel: 029 2037 1566
Fax: 029 2039 9562

Age Concern Northern Ireland
3 Lower Crescent
Belfast BT7 1NR
Tel: 028 9024 5729
Fax: 028 9023 5497

Other books in this series

The Carers Handbook series has been written for the families and friends of older people. It guides readers through key care situations and aims to help readers make informed, practical decisions. All the books in the series:

- are packed full of detailed advice and information;
- offer step-by-step guidance on the decisions that need to be taken;
- examine all the options available;
- are full of practical checklists and case studies;
- point you towards specialist help;
- guide you through the social services maze;
- help you to draft a personal plan of action;
- are fully up to date with recent guidelines and issues;
- draw on Age Concern's wealth of experience.

Already published

Caring for someone with an alcohol problem
Mike Ward
£6.99 0–86242–227–2

Caring for someone at a distance
Julie Spencer-Cingöz
£6.99 0–86242–228–0

Choices for the carer of an elderly relative
Marina Lewycka
£6.99 0–86242–263–9

Finding and paying for residential and nursing home care
Marina Lewycka
£6.99 0–86242–261–2

Caring for someone who has had a stroke
Philip Coyne with Penny Mares
£6.99 0–86242–264–7

Caring for someone with a heart problem
Toni Battison
£6.99 0–86242–252–3

Caring for someone who has dementia
Jane Brotchie
£6.99 0–86242–259–0

Caring for someone who is dying
Penny Mares
£6.99 0–86242–260–4

The Carer's Handbook: What to do and who to turn to
Marina Lewycka
£6.99 0–86242–262–0

Publications from Age Concern Books

Money matters

Your Rights: A guide to money benefits for older people
Sally West

A highly acclaimed annual guide to the state benefits available to older people. It contains current information on Income Support, Housing Benefit and retirement pensions, among other matters, and provides advice on how to claim.

For further information, please telephone 020 8765 7200

Managing Other People's Money, 2nd edition
Penny Letts

Foreword by the Master of the Court of Protection

The management of money and property is usually a personal and private matter. However, there may come a time when someone else has to take over on either a temporary or a permanent basis. This book looks at the circumstances in which such a need could arise and provides a step-by-step guide to the arrangements that have to be made.

£9.99 0–86242–250–7

Ethnic Elders' Benefits Handbook
Sue Ward

Written clearly and concisely, this book aims to help anyone from an ethnic minority understand how the Social Security benefits system works, what their rights are and how they can claim a benefit to which they may be entitled. It includes explanations of the legal issues covering immigration and citizenship.

£9.99 0–86242–229–9

Health and care

Know Your Medicines, 3rd edition
Pat Blair

The new edition of this handy guide explains many of the common questions older people – and those who care for them – may have about the medicines they use and how this may affect them. Topics covered include:

- what medicines actually do;
- using medicines more effectively;
- getting advice and asking questions;
- taking medicines safely;
- medicines and the body system;
- common ailments.

There is also information about the dosage and strength of medicines, brands, the storage and disposal of medicines, and an index to help look up medicines that are prescribed or bought over the counter. This new edition will serve as a valuable source of advice and guidance.

£7.99 0–86242–226–4

If you would like to order any of these titles, please write to the address below, enclosing a cheque or money order for the appropriate amount (plus £1.95 for postage and packing) made payable to Age Concern England. Credit card orders may be made on 020 8765 7200.

Mail Order Unit
Age Concern England
1268 London Road
London SW16 4ER

Information Line

Age Concern produces over 40 comprehensive factsheets designed to answer many of the questions older people – or those advising them – may have, on topics such as:

- finding and paying for residential and nursing home care;
- money benefits;
- finding help at home;
- legal affairs;
- making a Will;
- help with heating;
- raising income from your home;
- transfer of assets.

Age Concern offers a factsheet subscription service that presents all the factsheets in a folder, together with regular updates throughout the year. The first year's subscription currently costs £70. Single copies, up to a maximum of five, are available free on receipt of an sae.

> To order your FREE factsheet list, phone 0800 00 99 66 (a free call) or write to:
>
> **Age Concern**
> FREEPOST (SWB 30375)
> Ashburton
> Devon TQ13 7ZZ

Index